BEFORE YOU LEAVE!

An Intimate Peek Behind the Nursing Home & Assisted

Living Veil. Book II:

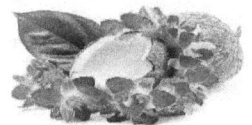

Larry D. Peden

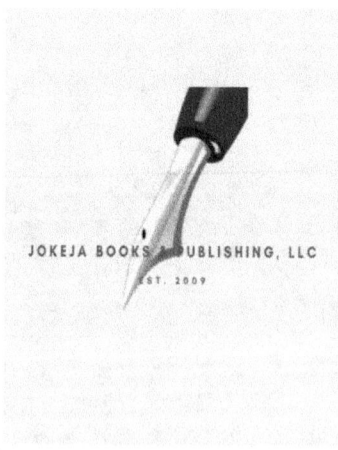

ACKNOWLEGMENTS

In loving memory of Kate; a remarkable woman, an enduring source of inspiration, a second mother to me, and an incredible friend. To my children, Joshua-Lawrence, KeishaElizabeth (Kebe), and Jason-James, you keep me sane. Thanks for patiently waiting for me to finish this thing. And to my grandchildren Jeremiah, Mariah, and Isaiah, who make me laugh more than should be legally allowed; behave, Grandma's watching!

And to my wife Evelyn, thank you! Your belief in me, has made it possible for me to become something more than I was. Nothing can change the gratitude I feel for having you in my life, and your love and support. You waited long and patiently for me to write this book. She was my best critic, advisor, and audience member as I recounted these stories. And special thanks to the various people I've shared these stories with over the past seven years: their keen interest showed me this was a book worth writing and one people were eager to hear. And special thanks to my co-workers in the geriatric nursing and assistance field, whose patience and mentoring helped me get through some extremely rough days. All of yo made this book possible, and I'm deeply grateful.

Finally, I want to thank Shirley, my dear friend, confidant, and former co-worker. Your insights and memory of events were immeasurably helpful in ensuring I did not miss anything, and it was cool hanging with you on the phone.

Edited By Dr. Lori Beth Sostock, MD

Family Medicine, Palliative and Hospice Care, Rush Medical College.

FORWARD

By Dr Barry Casey, Ph.D. Professor Emeritus, Department of Communications, Washington Adventist University, Takoma Park, Maryland. Retired.

"Don't get old, son," said my friend's elderly mother. "It's not for wimps." No, it is not, a fact that is attested to by Larry Peden's memoir of his years working in an assisted-living facility.

Through a combination of factors, Americans are living longer, but not better, lives. Vaccines in childhood, improvements in diet and exercise, better research, and an emphasis on preventative medicine have combined to increase life spans since the early twentieth century. But that also means that Americans who live longer than their grandparents did are spending more of those years slowly dying. Those who can afford it often end up in assisted-living facilities, where their physical and mental decline is accelerated by business practices that put money before medicine. Often, the Certified Nursing Assistants (CNAs) and the nurses are stretched to the limit because of understaffing, cost-cutting measures, and deceptive business practices.

Larry Peden has witnessed this firsthand in his years as a CNA. His story reveals the frustration, the heartache, but also the dedication of those who serve the elderly residents of these facilities. His books are not only a graphic day-by-day account of the trials and triumphs of such work, but also point the way forward through changes in policy. Larry Peden's account will open your eyes and break your heart.

Contents

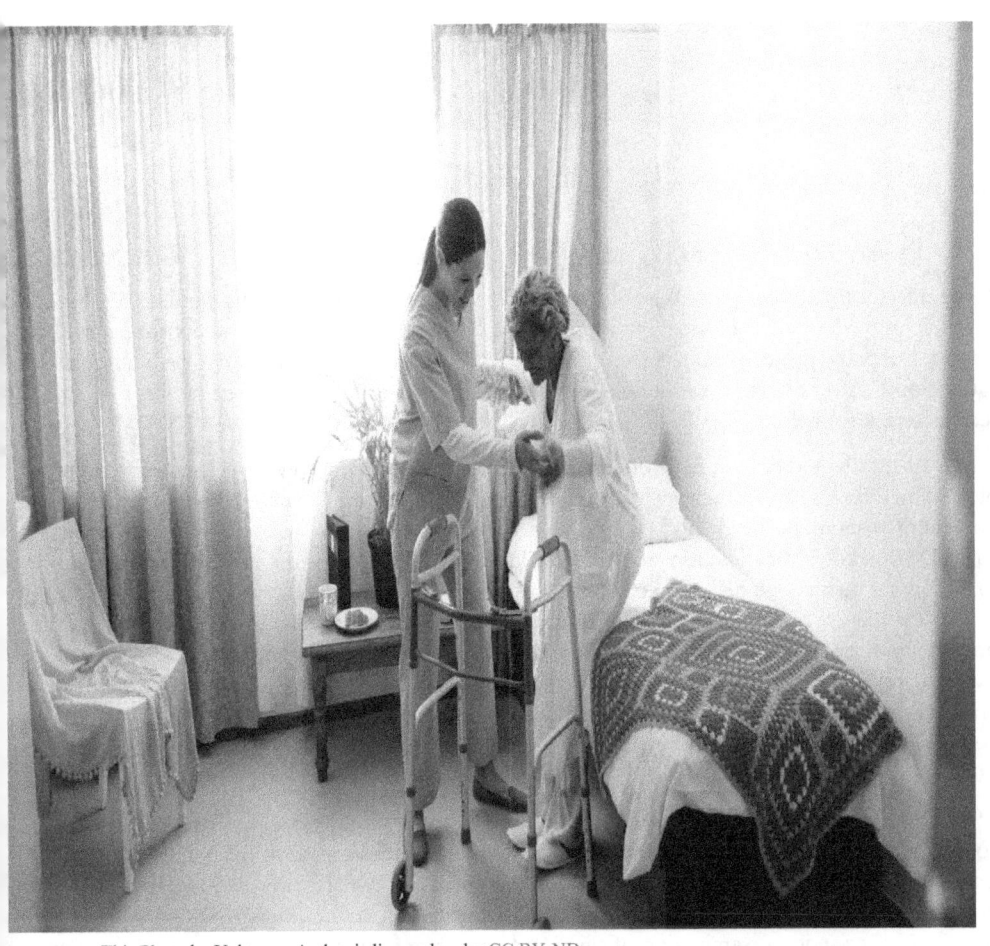

Introduction

Remembering my years in geriatric nursing, especially the first two years, reminds me of a story I once heard. A successful Wall Street investor went on vacation with his family. They headed down highway 95 towards Florida, but as they got into South Carolina they took a wrong turn and got lost. Despite repeated demands from the wife the husband continued to drive on, insisting, "I'll figure it out!" After driving for more than an hour he finally admitted to himself he was lost and decided to ask for help.

As luck would have it, he spotted an old farmer walking a mule heading towards. "Excuse me ole timer, do you know the way to Cornwall Road," he asked? The farmer thought about it for a moment then shook his head and said, "Nope, sorry I don't." "Well how about Solomon Wurth's Road? Do you know the directions to that," the investor asked? Again, the farmer thought about it for a moment then shook his head and said, "Nope, sorry I don't." "Well, how about Route 70? You've gotta know how to get to Route 70 from here," the investor yelled exasperated? The farmer thought about it for a moment then, then looked left then right, then shook his head and said, "Nope, sorry I don't." Angrily, the investor looked at the shabby dressed, and somewhat illiterate farmer and said, "You don't seem to know much of nothing about anything do you?" "The farmer looked down at the ground and thought about it, then looked up at him and said, "I know I ain't lost!"

You've made it to Book II, and that's proof you're not lost. You're in the right place. In Book I, you were introduced to the basic realities of the Geriatric and Certified Nursing Assistant profession, and the realities of long-term care in the nursing home and assisted living facility environment in America. Book II will take you deeper into that environment than you may want to go, but in any serious examination of aging and long-term care in the 21st century no sitting on the sidelines is genuinely safe or advisable. Things are about to get ugly. Pull up a seat!

PART I: NOTHING BEATS A GOOD SCANDAL

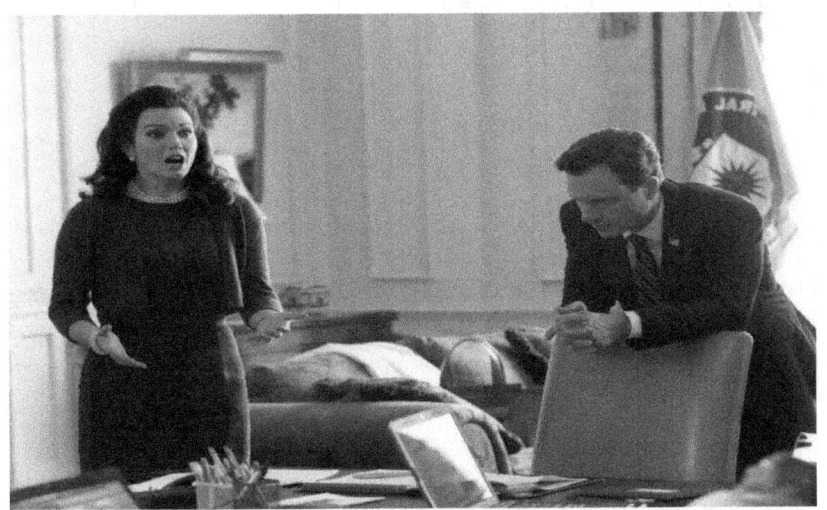

Noticeably absent from most Geriatric and Certified Nursing Assistant classrooms is the unmentioned, the things rumored, yet sometimes true, quietly kept out of the discussion. They are the things we hear about on the evening news and are shocked to learn, but already knew to be true from experience. Abuse, scandal, illegal practices and coverups, complaints voiced and quietly ignored, are sadly a very real part of the job in some situations, and any honest and serious discussion about the field must include them. Even though, to students, and patient's family it may be news.

DANCING IN THE FIRE

"From wrong to wrong the exasperated spirit proceeds, unless restored by the refining fire, where you must move in measure, like a dancer."

- T. S. Eliot

Not all patients are ready for a facility. Physically, they may need to be here, but mentally, they are not safe to be around. Sometimes they snap and violence is always a possibility. You get used to it to some degree, the possibility of violence: residents attacking the staff, residents attacking one another the staff attacking residents, and occasionally-if things get boring enough, staff attacking each other. Sooner or later, someone loses it. Geriatric nursing is not a spectator sport!

In the one and a-half years since I had been here much had not changed aesthetically. But now, the boring green couches and chairs were suddenly being replaced with newer, unstained, and greener couches and chairs free of odors, and the smelly green curtains succeeded by heinous beige ones. Filthy, broken square dining room tables were followed by cheap, decorative oval ones while drab white walls were repainted with fresh white paint. Except for the frequent hammering and occasional having to walk over a worker here or there most everyone barely paid any attention to what was going on or cared.   The ugly green carpet that had just been put in made me want to puck. It seemed so drab and out of place, clashing with the white walls and ambience of the building. When you stepped into the elevator the depressing unhomeliness was even more noticeable due to the smelly urine and vomit stains on the rug. Word was that management, having spent nearly fifteen thousand dollars to replace them, now, after the contractors had taking more than three months to install it while we worked around them, were ready to pull it all up and have a newer, costlier rug put down in its' place. It just seemed to magnify too much the ugly truth that this was a place where people came to die.

Sensing the mistake, management decided to spend a rumored two hundred thousand dollars more to completely remodel the whole place. Walking through the corridors, slogans painted on the walls, suddenly appeared. One got my attention, "The journey of a thousand miles begins with one step." "The facility can afford to spend two million dollars on renovations, but can't afford to provide adequate staffing," I thought to myself? "But then again, adequate staffing wasn't a priority, getting new clients was what matters."

It was a rainy Saturday afternoon, and the ride in had been pleasant, but within minutes I found myself circled by Shirley and Emily. Both visibly upset over what had happened overnight. Leo had wandered confusedly into Roberta's room during the night, and thinking she was an intruder sleeping in his bed, had demanded that she wake up and leave. Shocked, she screamed for him to get out, which enraged him, and he began beating her across her face and chest, as she fought back. Soon, the physical assault turned to sexual abuse as he ripped her night gown open and squeezed her hands so fiercely that they were sprained. Hearing the commotion, Shirley and Emily rushed into the room to help her and pulled Leo away from her. He swung hard at Shirley but missed. The momentum causing him to lose his balance and stumble. Helping him up from the floor, they quickly led him back to his room across the hall and got him to bed, then returned to check on Roberta, who Comfort stood over, checking her vitals, and trying to calm her.

Emily called Rhonda to report what had happed. It was standard procedure before calling the police. "Don't call them, I'm on the way" Rhonda ordered and hung up. With labored gestures and exasperated breathing, Emily and Shirley described the night's events to me, "He's got to get out of here. He almost killed her!" I headed upstairs to Roberta's room to check on her. She was in her bed staring at the wall angrily and her right eye was a bruised, black and blue, and her lip cut. "How are you Roberta," I asked quietly?

She looked at me briefly, then turned back towards the window and stared outside. Lifting her arm gently, I began to take her blood pressure and temperature and was horrified to see that both her hands were black and blue and bruised badly. Through the crevice of her gown I could see a huge chunk of her chest was also badly bruised. At her age, she was lucky to have survived such a beating. Eventually, she began to talk about the incident, struggling through tears to tell me what had happened. It was the same story I had heard from Shirley and Emily. When she had decided she had said enough, she reached for her walker and headed to the closet.

"What are you doing Roberta," I asked her puzzled? "You really should use your wheelchair. What are you up to?" She looked at me and pointed at the closet. "Get me that" she insisted! It took me a moment to realize that she was reaching for the golf club deep in the back. "What are you going to do with that," I asked her shocked? "I'm going across the hall and beat his damn skull in," she answered angrily!

After several minutes of calming her down, I talked her out of it and headed downstairs to notify Ishmael what had occurred. I was surprised to see Rhonda at the concierge's desk busy on the phone. Evidently, she had stayed all night after Leo's adventure, and was manning the phones for some reason, instead of hiding herself in her office as usual. I waited for her to finish.

"Is she going out to the hospital," I asked anxiously. "Who," she asked a little annoyed? "Roberta," I said. "Why does she need to go out to the hospital," she asked agitated? "Is something wrong with her?" "She's in her wheelchair, cursing about Leo and threatening to go into his room and kill him," I said!

"We're not going to send her out for something like that," she replied sarcastically. "Really!" "But she's upstairs with bruises all over her hands and face from where Leo attacked her," I answered, stunned by what I was hearing! "You don't know that," she argued back, "for all we know she might have slipped and fell and that's why she's bruised!"

I looked at her in amazement. She was serious. I took the elevator back upstairs to start my rounds. Less than an hour later, Charlene called me into her office. "What made you think it was your job to have someone sent out to the hospital," she demanded? "Your job is to notify your supervisor or me! Why did you tell Rhonda Roberta needed to go to the hospital," she scolded?

"She was bruised and crying when I checked on her," I explained, "and said she was in pain." "It's not your job to make those decisions," she continued to emphasis. "Her hands were black and blue," I interrupted, "and her eye was swollen!"

"Did you notify your supervisor," she demanded? "They were the ones who told me," I answered! "Told you what," she shouted?   "That Leo had attacked her," I blurted. "They told me what happened when I arrived."

"Nobody attacked anyone," she insisted. "You don't know what you're talking about." "The night shift stopped me this morning and told me what happened," I said, not wanting to name names. "But were you here at the time," she questioned?

"No, I was just going by what I was told," I answered. "See, there you go again, instigating things when you don't know what really happened," she shouted. "I'm not instigating anything. I'm going by what I was told me by the night shift," I told her again. "Plus, Roberta told me what had happened herself."

"You're instigating," she shouted again! "You're making accusations without any proof or facts!" "I'm not a cop, I'm not investigating anything," I said angrily! "I'm just reporting to you what I saw and what I was told, that's all!"   She looked at me angrily and shook her head and I could see that I was about to be blamed for something. The chewing-out by Charlene continued for another twenty minutes before I headed back to work. Later, as Shirley and I sat down to lunch, we talked about Rhonda and Charlene's reactions

"It doesn't surprise me, you know how they are," she retorted! "Charlene's a snake!" "This place is a lawsuit waiting to happen," I said angrily! "It really is!" "You don't know half the things that go on around here, especially the things that happened before you came here," Shirley said heatedly. "The State needs to come in here and really see what goes on, and how they really are. Somebody needs to fire their ass!"

"What they better hope is that Roberta's son doesn't come down unexpectedly. He's a lawyer, and he isn't going to buy their bullshit," I offered. "They can fool the State and everybody else, but he's going to want answers about what happened to his mother, and he's not going to be fooled by their crap." Fortunately for the facility, he lived several states away, was away on business often, and it would be several months before he stopped in again to see her. By then, the bruises would have vanished, Leo would have been quietly moved to another facility, and there would be no one to back-up Roberta's story if she complained to him, and he'd naturally attribute her complaining to dementia. But we all knew better.

Quietly, the facility slithered itself through this scandal unscathed then went back to business as usual, safe, and not under scrutiny. I put the incident behind me and tried not to think about it, and the violent outbursts residents were capable of, as the months went by. When I got home, I found a summons taped to our front door. It said *we owed seventeen hundred dollars, which must be paid by Tuesday, or they would take us to court to begin eviction proceedings*. "I hate my life," Rosa groaned, grabbed a pack of playing cards, and headed to the bedroom to be alone. "I should give this to Rhonda," I thought, "She's good at bullshitting people!"

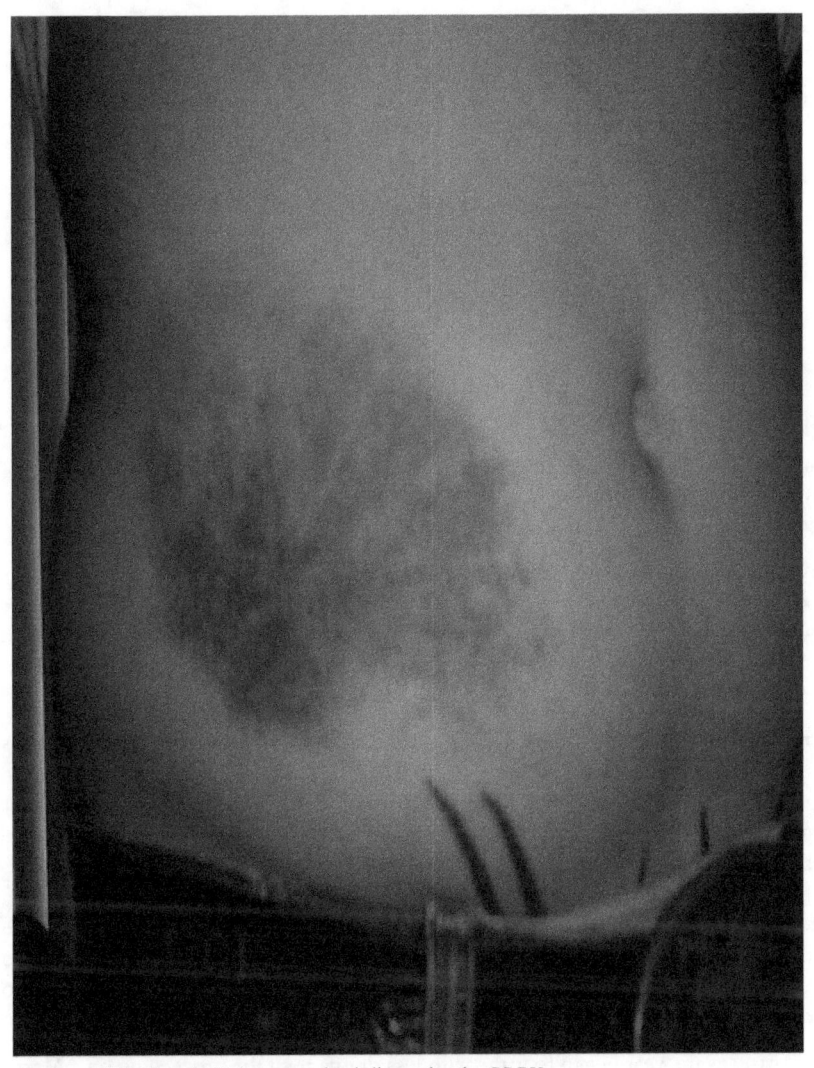

CIRCLING INSIDE THE MAZE

"Dying is a very dull, dreary affair. And my advice to you is to have nothing whatever to do with it."

- *Somerset Maugham*

Jamadar, we learned in school, had a master's degree in nursing, and was working on his Ph.D. A passionate Muslim, he sometimes, without warning, would suddenly burst out in an angry tirade, "I hate nursing. I cannot stand it. I can't take it another day," leaving us wonder what we were getting ourselves into!

I have never been nominated for Employee of the month. But lately, a lot of residents and co-workers had promised me their votes. "Everybody likes you," Kalie prodded me! "You help everybody with everything!" Finally, with my second year nearly over, after several folks promised me their vote, Marsalis, the kitchen worker won. Fixing broken appliances and peoples' cable connection could not compete with extra desert!

My relationship with Kalie had changed a great deal during the year. For a long time, she'd continued to dislike me, but gradually got use to my presence one month when she got extremely sick and stayed in her room. Concerned, I stopped by her room often to check on her, to make sure she was alright. When she was finally better, I continued to stop by and visit her, and during those times, we often talked and watched television together, as a close friendship developed. "The problem with you is that you don't know how to say no," she would scold me thoughtfully, after tiring of listening to me complain about my problems at home. "You're too nice! What, is she a princess?" She had that ability to buy past all my bullshit and put her finger right on the source of the problem. You have spoiled her, now you have a problem! Put your foot down and say no!" I wished it were that simple.

In any case, as the year began to wane with less drama than the proceeding one, Mary: a well-dressed, bossy, total care, paraplegic in her nineties, and her electric wheelchair-which she felt no one could maneuver properly, strolled in. I made sure she was my last patient of the evening, because of the enormous amount of time it would take to care for her. Everyone on the Nursing staff dreaded total care patients because they knew how much work was involved. With Mary, things took even longer. After thirty-five minutes of listening to her instruct me on how to do things before I got her into the bathroom, followed by thirty-five more minutes of getting her out-while she used the toilet and barked instructions on how to transfer her from the toilet to her wheelchair-I stood next to her waiting quietly and wondered why she always made something simple so complicated.

Behind schedule, I got her out of the bathroom and next to her bed. Lifting her from her wheelchair, I turned her around slowly and sat her down on it and lifted her feet so that she could lay back to get her diaper changed. Rolling her to one side, then almost to the edge of the bed to get it fastened without her falling onto the floor was more time than I wanted to spend caring for a resident, so when she was tucked safely in bed and the lights turned out, I hurried down the hall relieved.

In the lobby downstairs, I leaned back in the comfortable, brown, leather, recliner and enjoyed my diner and watched a good horror movie. I have noticed that the wealthier the resident, the more often relatives come by to visit. Visits are everything here. They keep residents safer, and staff less inclined to be callous or abusive. Well, up to a point anyway.

Sybil had arrived at the facility a few days ago. A quiet, friendly, short, elderly woman in her late eighties, who spent most of her time walking around investigating every inch of the place, she stopped to smile and greet everyone. At diner, she sat at her table and ate eagerly, and listened happily to the residents distribute the latest gossip. In the evenings, she headed upstairs to her room to watch television while she waited for a GNA to undress and put her in bed, which usually went very well: since she used the toilet on her own before retiring and woke up dry most mornings. This routine worked very well for the staff for the first four or five months, then things changed.

One day Ishmael found her wondering aimlessly in the hallway, completely oblivious to where she was or how to get back to her room. "Can you help me," she asked timidly, "I'm lost?" That was the beginning of her decline. Over the next few months, she became moody, more frequently confused and less communicative and willing to get out of bed. Still, she remained sweet, friendly, and cooperative whenever we changed her diaper or got her dressed, but something was a bit off deep inside her.

One day I walked in to find her daughter Nancy standing over her worried. She was trying to convince her mother to eat lunch, but it was not working. Bending closer to feed her a piece of toast, Nancy suddenly jerked backwards fearfully, which surprised me. "What's wrong," I asked puzzled?

"I can't get her to eat anything," she said in frustration. "Really," I said surprised? "She's always so friendly and funny whenever I take care of her." Nancy sat quietly and watched as I fed her mother breakfast, then said to me pensively, "She's really mellowed a lot I guess?" I asked her what she meant. "Growing up, she was always so strict and mean to me and my sister that we were afraid of her," she confided. "She wasn't a "so-sweet" woman before she got sick."

I thought it interesting how little we really knew about the people we took care of, caring for them at their most vulnerable moments, while assuming they lived charmed and blissful lives. Most had money. Many had had amazing careers. It had not occurred to me before, that their children paid the price for that success every now and then. Despite the past, Nancy visited her mother frequently each week, cleaning up behind her and tidying-up her room like a dutiful daughter, and took her for long walks outside whenever she could coach her to get out of bed. One day I walked in to find her standing over her mother's bed as she slept, looking down at her anguished and asked what was wrong. "She's sick and needs to go to the hospital, and I'm waiting for the administrators upstairs to okay sending her out," she said anxiously.

Realizing there was nothing more I could do, I wished them the best and left. Two weeks later, having already been rotated to another floor, by coincidence, I passed Sybil's room and saw Nancy sitting on the couch, and asked how her mother was. "She's in the bathroom, and she's getting worse" she told me sadly! "What did the doctors say," I asked her concerned? "What doctors," she replied?

"I thought she went to the hospital a few weeks ago," I questioned? "I keep asking them to call the doctor, but he keeps cancelling her appointments, and they won't send her out to the hospital," she said almost sobbing. "I'm really worried about her now!" Speaking quietly into her ear, I whispered to her, "That's your mother. If you called 911 or walked her downstairs to the car and took her to the hospital yourself, what could they do?" She looked at me surprised and asked, "Won't they get upset if I did that?" Putting my hand on her shoulder, I told her, who cares? If it were my mother, I wouldn't wait for them to get around to helping her!"

Minutes later, she and her mom were out the door, heading to the hospital. Less than a week later, she was back in her mother's room, collecting her things. "She died the second day at the hospital," she confided in me. They couldn't do anything. They kept telling me that if she'd just come in a few weeks earlier they could have saved her." We talked for a while about her mom, and she thanked and hugged me, then we said our goodbyes. That was the last time I saw her. I thought about it at times when I was changing resident's diapers. At work, I cared for thirty patients daily and kept all their idiosyncrasies in my head: their likes and dislikes, what made them angry and what worked, and seldom got it wrong, but the hardest task seemed to be seeing alternatives clearly, both for them, and my own life.

GRAPPLING WITHOUT A CONSCIENCE

"There is no good in arguing with the inevitable. The only argument available with an east wind is to put on your overcoat."

- *James Russell Lowell*

It has been a particularly hot summer this year, and often, I have found myself hard press to find enough shade outside to smoke a cigarette. One of the cooks, Cynthia-a pretty girl from Jamaica in her early twenties shocked me earlier, when she confided that she was punching off the clock so that she could go back to work inside. "That's illegal," I said to her bewildered, "why would you do that?

"What choice do I have," she replied angrily? "They know we don't have enough time to finish all of our work, but if we don't, they say we're not working hard enough and fire us!" "They can't force you to work for free, that's against the law," I insisted! "They can't do that!" "Well, they do," she answered angrily! "I'm not a citizen. I'm here on a green card, what can I do?"

"Did they order you to punch-out then return to work," I asked her? "No. They never tell you to, they expect you to," she answered! "They know that if you get off at three o'clock and you're still working at six, you're not on the clock." "And they don't say anything," I asked? "No. They leave you alone if you're off the clock and the work gets done," she persisted. "Sometimes, it's past seven when I get out of here, and I have to call a cab because I've missed my bus."

The halls have been quieter lately, due to the facility having lost so many residents because of deaths and move-outs. They have seemed more like ghost towns than dwelling places. You walk down them, and all you hear is the sound of a single television blaring somewhere in the distant corridor, and while it is nice not to be so busy, not being busy does not mean being overworked.

Paul and Thelma signed the paperwork weeks after Christmas, but waited until early February to move in. A short, Irish, and German couple in their early nineties, Paul clinging to his walker as though he feared it might get away from him, did all the speaking while she-suffering from stage four Alzheimer's disease, listened and complained constantly.

"Come on honey, let's go upstairs," he said to her gently. "They'll bring you something to drink in the room." "But why do I have to go upstairs," Thelma questioned puzzled. "I want to go home. When can we go home?" "We are home sweetie, how many times do I have to tell you," He answered her sharply? "Now, let's go upstairs."

"Why? Why can't we stay down here," she insisted confused? "Because this is the lobby, and we can't sleep here," Paul explained! The conversation continued for another four or five minutes, as he tried everything, he could think of to coach her into the elevator without success. Frustrated, he stepped inside, pressed the hold bottom, and yelled, "Are you coming, or aren't you Thelma?" Pouting, she walked inside and, stared quietly at the steel doors as they rode the elevator to the fourth floor, asking repeatedly, "When can we go home?"

For some unexplainable reason, the fire alarm has been going off frequently in the evening. There are planned fire drills that happen during the year. Each time, notices are placed around the facility to keep the residents from thinking a real fire is happening. Suddenly, the alarm lights started flashing and the doors to the corridors shut, to prevent a real fire from spreading, and a loud, shrilly noise sounded throughout the building piercing my ears and sanity, as Gary, the maintenance supervisor ran to the basement to shut it off.

Donna died in front of me this evening. Literally, just minutes after I walked into her room. She was another one of the new arrivals last year who made it in just as the wintry winds were beginning. A short, skinny, woman in her mid-nineties, with short gray hair and a friendly smile, she laughed and greeted people as her daughter pushed her in her wheelchair. I liked her immediately.

Years of smoking had done its damage though, and she had come here to die peacefully. Feisty, alert, and opinionated, she was quick to offer her views on anything someone wanted to talk about. During the three months she was at the facility, I became accustomed to stopping by her room regularly to chat and learn more about her. Even more, to learn about her daughter who was my age, divorced, well-to-do, and really cute-in a Demi Moore, Diane Lane sort of way. Like her mom, she had a gift for conversation, and was a defensive, die-hard football fan?

Her mom seemed as proud of her as she seemed devoted to her mother. The mutual affection between them was neither faked nor overly acted. The way they laughed and spoke to each other indicated that they were remarkably close, probably due to Donna being abandoned by her husband when Joanna was incredibly young. She had been instrumental in helping Joanna cope with her own ex-husband's infidelities.

When I walked into her room today to check on her, I was surprised to see her laying on her bed without a blanket, as the air conditioner blared. "Why are you lying here in the cold," I asked in amazement? She rolled over onto her back, looked at me and groaned, then stopped breathing. I moved closer to check her breathing. There was no oxygen coming or going her mouth or nostrils. No rising of the chest, or pulse. Lifting her eyelids, I checked for movement or signs of life. My visit had lasted less than three minutes, and it was the last one we would ever have. She was gone.

There are times when I really envy my patients though, when I wish I could be free from responsibilities like they are. Even though they are old and sick and waiting for death I long for the time when I am no longer burden with so many troubles. Their children are grown, their mortgages are paid, and all they really must do each day is wake up and keep breathing. There is a quiet sense of relief in that that I do not have. But not all of them are so free. Delores rolled into the facility around March. Feisty too and wildly alert, with a pleasant humor and friendly, she was more than eager to talk to the staff as they changed her diapers and clothes. Plus, she watched television constantly, which allowed me to catchup on what was going on in the world while we worked. At eighty-eight, she was tall, skinny, and-except for her feet, which were bent inwards and made it impossible for her to walk-she was in relatively good health. Always a plus. She had come to us from another facility forty miles away that she did not like too much, and immediately fell-in-love with the new carpeting and renovations that had been made.

Changing her diaper and pants as she lay upon her bed, then moving her to the chair was the normal routine we followed, before reaching for the clothes she had asked to have from her closet laid on the bed. Luckily, she had good taste, a sizeable wardrobe, and was not too picky if the pieces worked well together. As a young woman, she had taken a job with the government as a receptionist to do her part in assisting in the war effort. Afterwards, she had stayed on and worked herself up to the position of a transcriber, then later, assistant to her supervisor, even though as she put it, "I really did everything, because he didn't know his ass from his head, he was so dumb."

Her husband died when she was seventy-two, leaving her to care for one young, adopted daughter-the details of which, she would not explain even when asked, for some reason. For the most part, she blended well with many of the residents and formed a close friendship with three of the women who ate at the table she was assigned, and eventually becoming one of my major sources for keeping up with the latest gossip and rumors. "Have you heard anything about room one hundred and nine," she asked me one day? "I heard she went out to the hospital!"

"Not yet," I told her. "I'll let you know when I hear something." The residents knew more about what happened in this place than the administration and most of the staff. Despite efforts to hide the corpses when a resident died, they usually knew what had happened long before it was officially posted on the walls, and Delores was always one of those who seemed to know first. If two of the residents were indulging in secret liaisons or a love triangle, there was a good chance she and her girlfriends were already whispering about it to each other as they sat in the lobby watching and nodding to each other with laughter.

When she got a notice from the Administration office to either pay her rent or vacate in thirty days, even she was surprised by the news. She had always paid her bill faithfully from the money in her retirement fund, which was suppose too provide for her needs for several more years. But suddenly, and to her bewilderment, her checks had begun to bounce.

Through phone calls and letters from her bank, she learned that her Son-in-law and real daughter, who lived in her *'paid for'* house, had emptied her bank account and bought themselves a new truck and extra luxuries, leaving her broke.   "I'll move back into my house and put them out," she told me furiously. "I tell you; I've never trusted that man. I'd knock his head off his shoulders if he were here right now!"

Looking away, she turned towards the wall and sobbed, worried about what to do next while I continued to wipe her buttocks and fasten a fresh diaper, wondering how all this would turn out. After nearly two months of pleading and arguing with the facility administrators, she managed to convince them to let her stay while she threatened legal actions against her Son-in-law, Ricardo. He must have believed her, because he did whatever he needed to do, to come up with money each month as well as the back rent that was owed. Her love for the place waned somewhat after she was told 'the facility is a business, not a charity.'

As the facility again, got back to 'business as usual,' I was told to report to Paul and Thelma's room immediately. No details as usual, just to get there fast. Walking in, I could smell the fresh stench of feces even before I saw Paul standing next to the bed yelling at Thelma-who was backed into a corner-to change her clothes. "Hey babe, can you change her diaper for me," he asked frustrated?" "She stinks!"

He liked to refer to the GNA's as babe, in a kind of bebop tone that reminded me of those bearded beatnik poets you saw in New York night clubs in the sixties. You just got used to it after a while. Thelma, looking straight ahead as usual, eyed the opposite wall with fierce determination and declared, "I don't want to change my clothes and I don't want to go to bed!"

Word was that nighttime was Paul's time to have sex with his wife, something the Alzheimer's had made easier for him to do regularly, and he had seldom missed a night since they had moved in.

"I'll take care of it," I told him. Moving towards her, I could see feces covering the floor and the wall behind her. After nearly forty minutes of coaching and diverting her attention, I managed to get her cleaned, dressed and in bed, so that Paul could 'sleep,' then spent another fifteen minutes cleaning her wall and rug.

Once a year it seems, some bad-ass virus works its way through the facility and makes a lot of people sick. Last year, it was the flu. I forget what, the year before that. This year, being so busy, I chalked it up to flu again and kept moving. My mistake. This year's malady seemed to be a gastrointestinal virus making its way across the country. Broadcasters mentioned it frequently on the news for weeks.

The leaves on the trees had already turned red, as fall settled in early in September. The constant flow of people visiting and residents leaving to visit family had made the facility a fertile roadway for the virus to travel and thrive as resident after resident and their relatives became infected. Recognizing something was happening, the administrators moved quickly to quarantine the sick and limit them to their rooms, and to put up posters warning visitors to wash their hands and to stay away if possible.

As the virus continued to work its way through the halls of the building, the GNA staff was given the additional duty of bringing and retrieving each residents' meals daily. To make matters worse, the elevators, for some reason, broke down frequently during those weeks, and we found ourselves making endless trips up and down the steps to all the floors to ensure everyone got fed. Finally, after the fifth week, the virus seemed to be slowing down, and everyone who was going to catch it, had. Well, almost.

Riding down the elevator that had finally been fixed for the second time in the week, as I covered the tray of food in front of me and waited for the elevator to reach the first floor, a searing pain shot through my abdomen. I almost buckled in agony wondering what was happening as a strong sense of nausea swept over me. When the doors opened, I headed towards the dining room with a pain in my body running from my stomach into my legs and feet. By the time I had made it back to the elevator, walking and standing had become unbearable. I hurried to the bathroom and vomited.

Charlene was not totally unsupportive when it became clear I would be out for a few days, but she was not particularly happy about it either. "We'll get by somehow," she said reluctantly as I headed downstairs to my car. "Hope you feel better!" Two days later I was at my doctors' office asking for an antibiotic and something for the pain. "Do you have a history of kidney disease in your family," he asked to my surprise? "Not that I know of," I answered.

"I want to send you to a renal specialist to be checked out just in case," he cautioned and handed me a referral. "My father had a kidney transplant a few years ago," I informed the specialist, "but he uses to drink all the time." "I need you to have some blood work done, then return to see me again afterwards," he answered pensively. "Just routine."

He gave me the bad news a week later, "You have polycystic kidney disease, a digressive disease that causes porous cists to form on your kidneys. There is no cure, but with medicine to control your blood pressure, and diet, the progression can be slowed down, but ultimately, you'll need a kidney transplant or dialysis."

Charlene took the news better than I did, relived that I was back to work and planned to stay busy. Luckily, the work offered little opportunities for me to reflect or be depressed over the death sentence hanging over me as I poured myself into caring for my residents. Apart from the usual annual training in Cardio-Pulmonary Resuscitation (CPR), first-aid, Alzheimer's and dementia care, hazardous material handling and fire safety drills which we muddled through year after year, this year, the facility brought in a nurse from the Board of Nursing to update us on the latest procedures and techniques for caring for our residents and to keep our licenses valid.

As she reviewed current trends and practices and tested us on them- a great way to spend an hour-and-a-half, Oulu asked about an issue that he seemed to disagree with her on. Sensing that she was not getting through to him and tiring of the debate, she changed the subject to patient suicides and asked innocently, "How many of you have had patients try to commit suicide?"

My hand shot up. Rhonda looked at me disapprovingly and nodded her head angrily as she asked the question a second time. "There have been no suicides here," she said to the instructor, "we don't have that here…"

Thinking of Charlie, and a few other residents, I stopped her and said, "I can think of at least three residents who did." "If someone committed suicide or we thought someone was going to do so we would be obligated to report it to the police," Rhonda emphasized to the class and looked at me annoyed. "Accusations and rumors are not proof, so let's not talk about things we can't prove."

I could feel her eyes watching me as the class began to end, and just like that, I was back in hot water with the administration, having broken the most sacred of the unwritten rules: see no evil, hear no evil, and never speak about anything to outsiders.

Barely out the room, had I received a call to report to Charlene's office? She was livid. "What makes you think you can make wild accusations about what goes on here? You haven't been here long enough to know what does or doesn't happen," she snapped!

"What are you talking about," I asked, surprised at her rage? "Where do you get off telling people someone committed suicide here," she scolded me like I was a little boy?

"I was just answering a question," I answered. "Everyone here knows Charlie and some residents starved themselves to death." "How do you know that," she demanded? "Did you see him do it, and if so, did you report it?"

"Charlene, I told you many times that Charlie refused to eat, and that he said repeatedly he was starving himself and wanted to die. I even wrote it in the logs that he refused to eat daily for months, and of another resident who did the same."

"We have legal regulations we have to follow," she insisted! "You don't make false accusations like that, ever! No one here is ever committed suicide. Got it?" "Now I've got to figure out what to do with you," she shouted furiously!

"I just answered the woman's question," I said sheepishly, and headed back downstairs to work, wondering if I was going to be fired or suspended. Neither as it turned out, but neither Charlene nor Rhonda spoke to me for nearly two weeks. I went home and iced down my knee, which had begun to swell because of the calcium build up in my kneecap, noting that my kidney disease was getting worse.

PART II: ALL GOOD THINGS

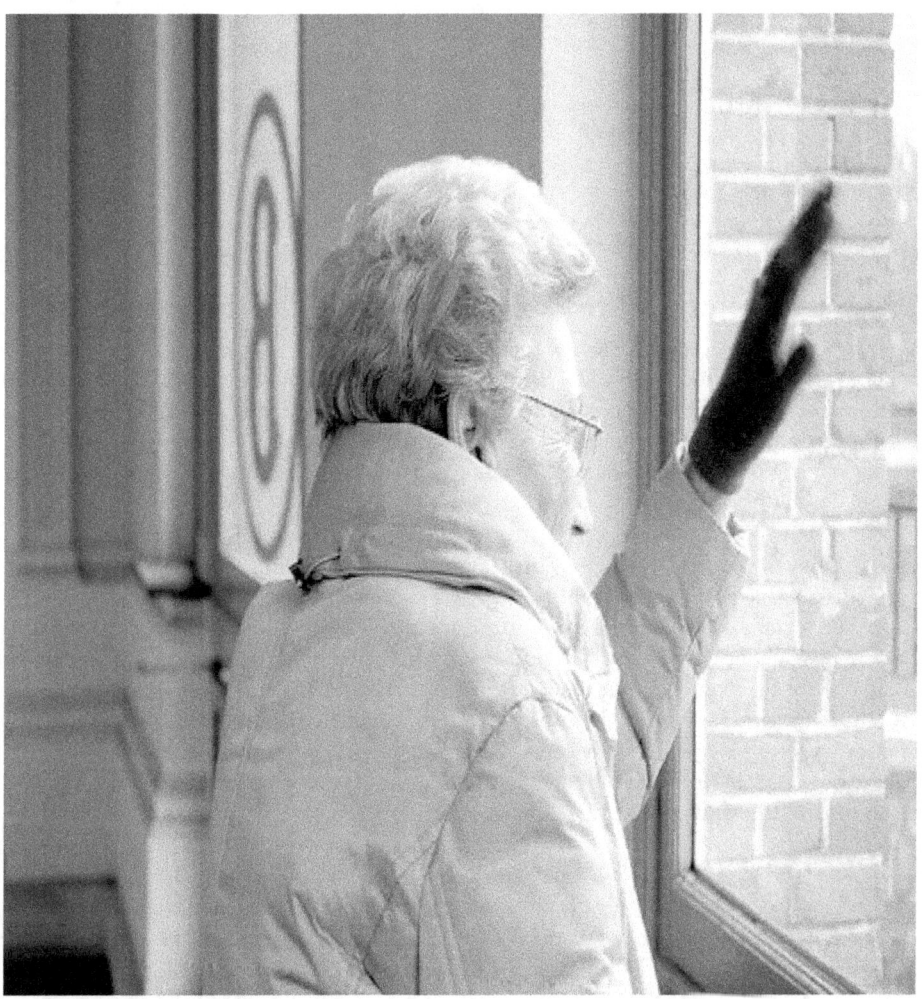

WHEN THE GLASS CRACKS

"I was so tired of the parts I had to play."

- *Anna May Wong*

So, this polycystic kidney disease is slowly killing me. That sucks, to have no real control over where the disease carries me month from month! I used to spend so much time worrying about my patient's future, now I am worrying more and more about my own. I didn't worry about death before, now, I think about it all the time, and the challenge to stay alive, with the barrage of pills, appointments, exercise, and relentless watching of my diet that I'm trying to get used to. I'm already missing the days when nausea, vomiting, stomach pains, and painful gout weren't the norm, but life doesn't stop because you get sick.

Life went on for Delores too, after months of haggling with administrators over her payments being late, with her daughters' help, she packed her bags and moved to a less expensive facility a few miles away. To everyone's surprise and relief, Beverly chose to depart the facility alsoand this life-during those non-eventful days, that Delores was moving out. "The snake lady is gone too," I heard someone joke behind me as I watched the men in black take her out! I turned to see who it was applauding, but they were gone. It sounded like Emily, but I could not be sure. And life continued to go on, the elderly kept coming and the sick kept dying, while management kept collecting rent and fees for just about everything, as we kept moving from room to room one diaper at a time, and I slowly got sicker.

I always suspected my job would end just as abruptly as it had begun, and it was inevitable that another violent attack would occur. On a sunny but cold evening in November, Mason arrived, and we were all relieved that he was in his right mind. A large, black man in his eighties, he was polite, friendly, and obviously had managed to be quite successful throughout his life-the type of someone use to talking to people from all walks of life and knew how to make you feel comfortable. More importantly, he was cooperative and kept a tidy, sparsely furnished and uncluttered room, and he did not mind being told what to do.

His family seemed friendly too, though a bit stand-offish. They respected the staff and the work we did and did not get in the way. "Diner time," I told him politely sticking my head through the door to see him sitting upon his couch talking to his wife and son, "See you downstairs."

"Where do I go," he asked me smilingly and stood? "Take the elevator to the first floor and turn to your left," I answered, closing the door behind me. "I'll be right down," I heard him say, and went down the hall to fetch more residents. That went well," I thought to myself, relieved to have someone normal on the floor again. "He'll be here for at least a year or two!"

Residential rentals had been down fifty percent for quite a while, and management had for some time solicited people in all kinds of health conditions with little regard to how the increased workload would burden the nursing staff. Basically, if they could make it through the door still breathing and could pay, they were accepted. Terminal cancer patients with just months to live; double amputees with diabetes and heart disease; stage six Alzheimer's disease folks who didn't know their own names anymore or anyone else's: if the money was there, they were ushered in happily and assigned a room, the ink on their leases barely dry before some of them expired, and their families returned to collect their belongings.

"You think they're going to wash all those behinds," I quipped to Lawrence. "Don't be ridiculous," he fired back, "If one of them residents pissed on Rhonda's shoe, she'd be calling us to come wash it off!" We laughed and headed to the dining room. I had dining room duty again and the task of jotting down who was eating, and how much. Soon it would be snack time and time to get the residents to bed, then relax. Luckily, Martha wanted to go to bed around nine-thirty, which meant I would get an hour of peace before I went to take care of her.

Sitting in the lounge watching television, the thought of my mother working as a maid to pay for college to escape poverty flashed through my mind. She had come from a backward scarcity that no longer existed in America and had sacrificed to give herself and her children a better future, and here I was, a college graduate, working as a medical maid. The contrast was painfully humiliating, and as I bent down to pick up a piece of paper my cell phone fell out my pocket.

Picking it up, I was about to put it back into my pocket when Matilda-a MedTech who had started working here just two days ago, shouted my name. Turning to see what she wanted I saw Mason standing over me. He mumbled something I could not make out then looked at me angrily and violently snatched the phone from my hand. I yelled for him to give it back. Instead, he looked at the phone, then at me, and began banging it against the wall, cracking it.

"Stop it," I yelled at him in shock, worried that he would somehow destroy the pictures I had just taken of my daughter and grandson. Realizing it bothered me, he backed away and looked at me, then began smashing the phone more. I moved towards him angrily, trying to figure some way to get him to stop. He turned and walked away, banging the phone into the walls repeatedly as he retreated. Seeing me in pursuit behind him, he turned to face, and clenched his fist in defiance.

"Give me back my phone," I shouted, almost tearfully! Then he punched me in the face. It did not hurt much, but it made me wonder what else he was capable of and how far he would take things before this was over. "Give me back my damn phone," I demanded, "right, fucking now!"

Mason grabbed a nearby broom that the House keeping department had left out accidently and swung it at my head. Realizing he had missed, he lunged forward and swung again, but missed. I pushed a nearby chair in front of him, to give myself distance, and grabbed a pair of scissors from the Concierge's desk and waved it in front of me to deter him. He backed away angrily and began pacing back and forth in the lobby. "You really need to go to your room sir," I said nervously. "They need to get you the hell out of here!"

He continued his pacing for several minutes, then without warning, started turning the furniture over, first a chair, then a couch, then a table. Seeing a small vase on a nearby end-table, he grabbed it and flung it at the glass doors. A huge crack appeared where the vase had struck. Upset that it had not broken, he ripped a leg from the table and began banging the glass hard, which only made the crack larger and created more cracks.

Realizing that he could not break the glass, he headed towards the corridors. Suddenly, my fears of being harmed shifted to fear of him hurting the residents: what would happen if he got into their rooms, in his agitated state, and the damage that he could do. "If he gets into one of those rooms, he could kill somebody," I said to myself! He had to be stopped, immediately.

I ran ahead of him and cut him off before he had a chance to reach a corridor. He was incensed. Holding the broom over his head, he began swinging it wildly at me, to get by. I slashed at the air in front of him angrily. He backed away. The minutes felt like hours as I pursued him all the way to the glass doors, hoping to somehow get him outside of the building, then deal with him there. We were still engaged in this "slash and swing" struggle, when the red and blue siren lights of a police car out front caught my attention. Then my hand exploded in pain. Mason had used the distraction to knock the scissors from my hand. Picking them up, he stood in front of me waving them at me and cursing.

"I need you to put down the scissors right now," the officers shouted! Mason looked back and forth, between them and me, and pointed the scissors menacingly. "What's wrong with him? Is he on medication," one of the officers asked me?   "I don't know," I answered him. "He's only been here a few days. I don't know what's wrong with him!"

"Sir, I need you to put down the scissors right away…," the officer repeated. "Or what…," Mason cut him off? "What the hell you gonna do if I don't? "Then we're going to have to restrain you sir, if you don't cooperate," the officer replied. "You ain't restraining me mutafuckas," he shouted and moved towards the officers. "You ain't gonna do a mutafucking thing to me!"

They backed away. Mason cursed and taunted the officers repeatedly for several minutes, leaning forward several times, as though he was trying to reach their guns. "I'm a mutafucking marine got dam it! You ain't gonna do a damn thing to me. You sons-of-a-bitches!" One of the officers reached for his gun, while the other reached for his Taser as Mason made a feeble attempt to lunge forward, but the officers put up their arms to block him, then both reached for their guns. Mason stepped back, to retreat inside, but tripping over his own feet slipped, and fell hard on the lobby floor. Seizing the opportunity, the officers jumped on him, before he had a chance to recover and get back up. As he pushed and struck out at the officers as they struggled to turn him onto his stomach, I grabbed his outstretched arm and bent it behind his back, to give the officers the leverage they needed to restrain him. "Yeah, you fucked-up now, didn't you," I smirked! Snatching my phone from his hand finally, I screamed at the officers, "Get him the hell out of here!"

Matilda tapped me on the shoulder and handed me her cellphone. "It's Charlene," she said nervously! She was furious. "Who told you to call the police<" she screamed! "How many times have I told you, if there is a problem, call me? What have you done this time?" I let her vent before explaining the situation, but she was not interested in the details, just that the police where present and that the family would have to be notified.

"He really tore the place up," I continued. "When I saw, he was determined to make his way down the hallways, I knew I had to do something to protect the residents." "Where was Ishmael? Why didn't you call him for help," she demanded? "You guys are a team; you're supposed to work together!" "I don't know where he is," I answered her. "I was too busy trying to keep that crazy fool from killing somebody, to look for him."

"What did you do," she demanded, "how did all this happen? "I didn't do anything," I explained. "I was sitting in a chair in the lobby watching television when Matilda suddenly screamed my name. When I looked up, there was Mason standing over me. It's all on tape." "Well, what were you doing in the lobby watching television," she demanded. "You always do this," she shouted. "You upset these residents, you rile them up, then run at the first sign of trouble..." Her words stung like a punch in the throat because I knew where all of it was heading and that she had already made up her mind that I was to blame for all that had happened.   "I quit! I've had enough of this, bullshit," I yelled, cutting her off! "I'm done!" Handing the phone to one of the police officers, I said, "this crazy bitch wants to blame me for all of this. Here! You talk to her, explain what happened here. I quit!" He took the phone from my hand and the two of them talked, as I turned and headed downstairs to my locker. The harsh tone in Charlene's voice told me it was time to leave, and that it was over as far as I was concerned.

Realistically, things were just beginning. I had tired of putting myself in harm's way and cleared out my locker and walked out into the cold night, angry and afraid. "What would become of them," I wondered? "What would become of me? Suddenly, after nearly four years, I was unemployed again!"

24

DROPPED FRUITS

"Overhead, overhead

Rushes life in a race,

As the clouds the clouds chase;

And we go,

And we drop like the fruits of the tree,

Even we,

Even so."

- *George Meredith*

In the end, Rhonda and Charlene did what I had pretty much expected them to do and implied that I had somehow caused Mason's violent outburst and was of course responsible for the situation getting out of control. Luckily, I knew the security cameras-if they were working, would back up my story, despite their accusations. Fortunately, they were, and there was no way for them to wiggle out of it as they had done so many times before. There would be an investigation, and this time no one to pen it on. I imagine both got little sleep for several weeks.

I spent the next several days trying to defend my actions to representatives from the Unemployment office while the facility affirmed repeatedly that, "they provided adequate training and support to keep such incidents from occurring, but that, if and when such incidents did occur, it was rare and clearly due to the actions of an employee, not the patient or facility itself."

This expected bullshit they managed to reiterate repeatedly for a while until someone at the facility screwed-up magnanimously, because months after I'd left, Banta told me over the phone, that now each floor provides a minimum of two GNA. To everyone's amazement the State had been there four times in the months immediately after I had left, to inspect without prior notification. Something unheard of! In the years I was there they seldom came more than once a year and always with prior notification. But now, as she struggled to get it all out, things had changed dramatically after at least six residents had died, and three of those deaths had been highly suspicious. So much in fact that Charlene had been fired amid allegations that a GNA had beat a resident so severely he died a week later, that had had reached the State Board of Nursing. It seemed the truth was unravelling its own path into the open, while commercials promoting the facility continued to run on the television.

Roberta, to the relief of some, also died suddenly. Apparently, by natural causes. Perhaps, out of sentiment rather than habit, her son began to come by the facility to visit the residents each month, but the facility viewed it as trespassing, and demanded he cease. "Your mother's dead, you don't have a reason to be here anymore," they complained bitterly! He stopped soon afterwards. Then Banta told me the sad news of how Kalie also had gotten sick and died after I'd left, and I couldn't help but feel guilty, and that somehow, I had let her down.

As I said from the beginning, the elderly is America's emerging majority race, an 'easily forgotten' and rapidly growing culture, and the most in danger of abusing and being abused. The harsh reality of aging is that it is often quite ugly, and most of us are not prepared for it, and many of us will spend our final days in some type of facility regardless of what kills us, surrounded by an ever-shrinking pool of qualified professionals to care for us. As I stated earlier, it has been estimated that more than sixty percent of the population will be over sixty in the next forty years. Geriatric Nursing is a field like any other, filed with good people and good intentions, and those unwilling to see the problems right in front of them. And there are even good facilities out there that do not turn a blind eye to things, and much that can be done to protect both patients and staff.

During my years in nursing, I watched my finances dwindle, my health frequently wane, and my marriage struggle, and thought often about writing this book and what I would say. Now that I am on dialysis and my fruit has begun to fall, I have the time and the task has taken on new meaning. I look back at that time with both fond and bitter memories, and utter surprise at my ability to love beyond what I thought I was capable. Undoubtedly, this book will raise some eyebrows and criticism, but nothing in these pages, except the actual names have been fabricated. I owed that to Kalie, and Fred, and Shelly, and the so many of my patients whose voices at times were ignored by those who should have been listening. I still do, and their voices, "being dead still speaks!"

CONCLUSIONS

Geriatric and Certified Nursing Assistance is a noble profession, and those that enter it must be of the highest character. I believe most are. It begins with unfamiliarity and uncertainty, and fear of the job, the patients, and one's ability to succeed, and progresses to learning the job, patients, and environment. Along the way you discover fatigue, violence, scandals, and turnover. You discover staff aren't always all they should be, and that patients don't necessarily get along, or get the best care because they're in a facility. The field by nature brings out the best in some, and the worst in others, and often requires great sacrifice on the part of those who enter it. Yet, never has the need for good people to enter it been greater. And that need is increasing with every approaching decade.

The big challenge of the 21st century in America is to find people qualified and willing to care for the aging and diverse American population that's here already and coming. The COVID pandemic has highlighted the healthcare disparities among whites and minorities, and for the firsttime real changes in healthcare are being talked about in government and the healthcare industry. Across the country people are realizing the current models aren't working or feasible for the years ahead. Not surprisingly, nursing homes suffered the most devastating casualties during the pandemic, and we watched in horror as they were powerless to save the lives of their patients, or their own. And with more pandemics coming the need for more people to enter the geriatric and certified nursing profession continues to increase.

The decades ahead will require healthcare professionals who understand that the care of our elderly and sick isn't a business, it's a responsibility, and it must be one they're willing to undertake. The challenge is daunting. In less than twenty-five years sixty percent of our county's population will be over sixty. And a sizeable percent of that population will need long-term care, which means that less than forty percent of the population will be available to provide it. Among that forty percent will come our future geriatric and certified nursing assistants who have stepped up to the plate. This book, and the book that preceded it will hopefully go far in helping you and them to prepare for that future to come. Hopefully.

PART III: SUPPLEMENTAL READINGS FOR FURTHER THOUGHT

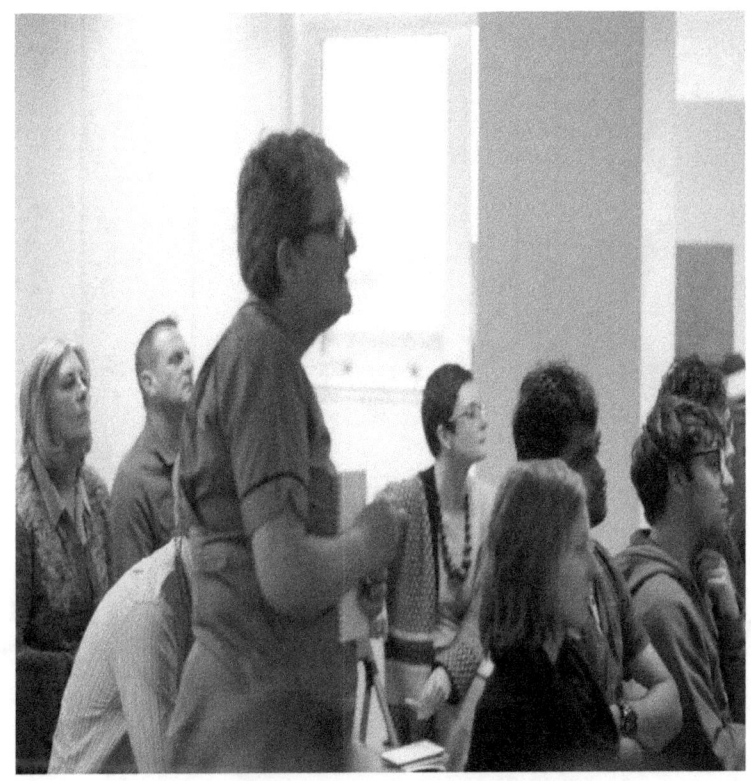

This Photo by Unknown Author is licensed under CC BY-NC

Proceeding Reading Material:

A: Building an Aging Agenda for the 21ˢᵗ Century

B: Family and Elder Care in the Twenty-First Century

C: Why a Family Support System is Important for the Elderly

D: Health and Aging in the 21st Century

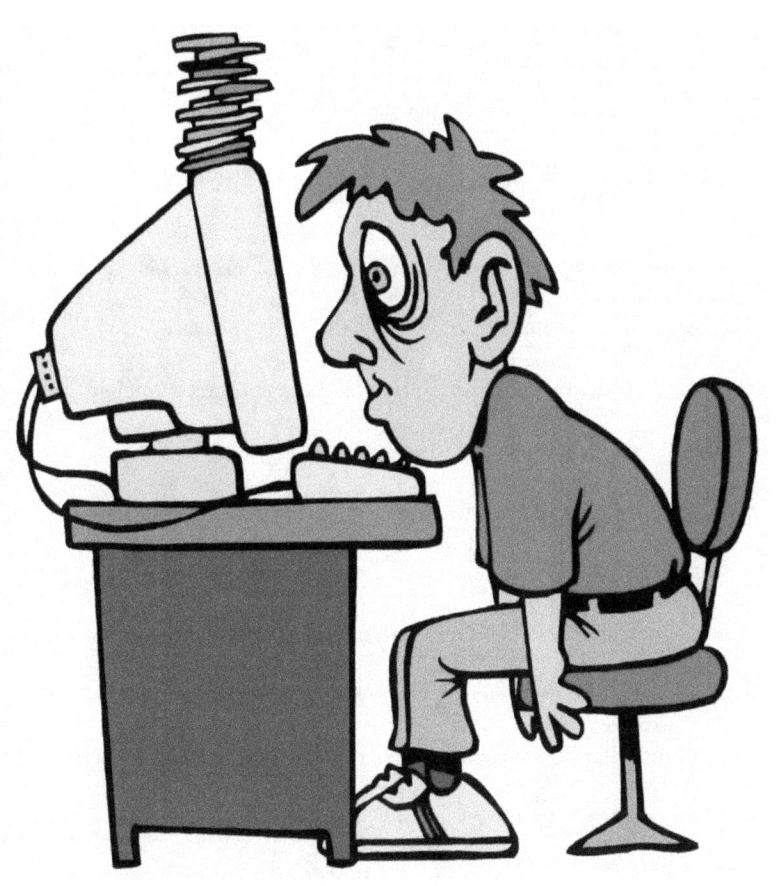

Excerpts from:

A   Building an Aging Agenda for the 21st Century

Building an Aging Agenda for the 21st Century During the next ten years, we have a window of opportunity to prepare for a dramatic "graying" of the state's population. This demographic shift will be felt across the board, from housing and transportation to civic planning and health services.

Many of these challenges are already upon us. We have a fragmented network of services that is stretched beyond its capacity. We face an unprecedented growth in the aging population, yet we continue to face critical budget crises at the state and national levels that threaten the core of services essential to keeping the senior population in their homes and communities.

Policymakers and advocates have been trying to fix the system for the past 20 years. A laundry list of reforms has been proposed by the Assembly Committee on Aging and LongTerm Care, the Little Hoover Commission and the Legislative Analyst's Office. Some have been enacted. But the pace of change has been slow, and it has never been directed by a single road map.

This is not good enough. Older Californians deserve better. We need to have a single plan to address the problems plaguing our system. I have been working on this singular vision since I became Chair of the Assembly Committee on Aging and Long-Term Care. It is my hope that this report

California has been a national leader in change in many areas, from air quality standards to civil rights. It's time that we approach our system of care and services for older adults and people with disabilities with the same level of determination and innovation.

This report will establish a policy roadmap as we begin to prepare California to meet the needs of older adults and people with disabilities today, and tomorrow. Change is never easy, but it's certainly not impossible. Let's build our vision together and move California forward.

-Assemblywoman Patty Berg

In the spring of 2004, Assemblywoman Patty Berg, Chair of the Assembly Committee on Aging and Long-Term Care, convened three committees to develop a Master Plan on Aging. The first of the three committees, the Strategic Plan Advisory Committee, further refined the priorities in the Strategic Plan for an Aging California Population (SB 910 [Vasconcellos], Chapter 984, Statutes of 1999) to the emerging trends most likely to result in fundamental systemic reform to the State's current service delivery system for older persons. The second committee, the Expert Panel to Review the California Department of Aging, responded to the call for reform regarding the administration of aging and long-term care services at the state level. The third committee, the Committee to Advance an Aging Agenda for the 21st Century, sought to develop legislative priorities, and strategic grassroots implementation steps based on the emerging trends to move an aging agenda forward. The Master Plan on Aging represents the efforts of experts from across the aging community, brought together in an effort to help guide policymakers and stakeholders as they develop comprehensive and meaningful legislative, grassroots, and policy agendas to address the issues surrounding the aging of California's baby boomers. In advancing the aging agenda, strong leadership will produce numerous future dividends for virtually all segments of our society.

California has more people who are age 65 and older than any other state, and the number is expected to grow dramatically in the years to come, with most of the growth predicted to occur between 2010 and 2030. By the year 2020, the number of people in California age 65 and older is projected to nearly double to more than 6.5 million. Conservatively, this will represent approximately 14 percent of California's total population. The greatest growth within the older population will be among the oldest Californians, those age 85 and older. By 2030, this population cohort will constitute one in five of the state's older residents. As California ages, it is becoming more racially and ethnically diverse, surpassed only by Hawaii. The state's aging population is expected to become even more diverse during the first half of the 21st century. More than 40 percent of baby boomers are African American, Latino, or Asian, and one third were born outside of the United States.

California is at a crossroads. Assembly Committee on Aging and Long-Term Care Assemblywoman Patty Berg, Chair Contributors Dixon Arnett Pauline Abbott Joaquin Anguera Dion Aroner Ann Burns Johnson Ronald Lee Ray Mastalish Erin O'Keefe Tom Porter Andrew Scharlach Steve Schmoll Peter Spaulding Fernando Torres-Gil Staff Allison Ruff Sarah S. Steenhausen 1020 N Street Suite 360 Sacramento, CA 95814 (916) 319-3990 September, 2006 **Four components have been identified as critical for the progressive change needed to enable California to effectively serve its current population of older adults, and prepare for the aging baby boomers. These components include a restructuring of aging and long-term care services at the state level; an integrated approach to data collection; an adequately trained workforce for service delivery; and the development of a coordinated grassroots advocacy network.**

Despite California's array of home and community-based services, multiple funding streams and varied eligibility criteria have created "silos" of services, making it difficult for consumers to move with ease from one service or program to another. The delivery of home and community-based services needs to be vastly improved in order to coordinate services that are appropriate to each individual's functional needs and financial situation. Establish a preadmission screening process to prevent unnecessary nursing home utilization.

- Develop and implement a uniform assessment tool for all home and community-based services for older adults and adults with disabilities to reduce duplication and fragmentation as consumers utilize multiple services and programs.

- Restructure the administration of long-term care programs at the state level, utilizing an organizational plan that incorporates sound business practices with broad governmental oversight and consolidates home and community-based services for older adults and people with disabilities under one administrative umbrella (See Restructuring the California Department of Aging and Long-Term Care Services in California report).

During the next 10 years, the state must prepare for the changes that will affect virtually every aspect of life: economic growth, housing and transportation systems, geographic and landuse planning needs, health and social services, and a host of public and private sector concerns. California will need to reevaluate the adequacy of current policies and systems of delivering services to meet the needs of the aging population, especially in light of increasing diversity[1].

In order to serve older adults and people with disabilities in an effective and efficient manner, the data collection system used by the variety of service providers and administrative entities needs to evolve. The current system reflects the fragmentation in the administration of programs, with different service providers collecting and reporting different information regarding individual service usage. Although many individuals use a variety of community-based services, California does not have a uniform system that would allow for tracking an individual across programs. The current system inhibits care navigation for providers and consumers alike and fails to meet federal and state regulations for data collection.

The development of an integrated data system would also enable a statewide care navigation system. With adequate, real-time data, the navigation system would enable consumers and providers to access a databank web site that provides a specific inventory of services for each county, with eligibility, application information online, as well as shared provider client tracking abilities. Similar database websites already exist but have not yet been developed on a statewide basis. These data systems help to reduce administrative inefficiencies and duplication in services.

The aging of California will increase the demand for professionals with expertise in the aging process. At present, California faces a severe shortage of professionals and paraprofessionals needed to operate programs and provide services for older adults. There

---

[1] Scharlach, A.; Torres-Gil, F.; Kaskie, B. (2001). *Strategic planning framework for an aging population*. California Policy Research Center

are approximately 890 board-certified geriatricians in the state: one geriatrician per 4,000 Californians age 65 and older. In addition, 62 percent of licensed social workers have or have had care management responsibilities, yet only 5 percent have received any social work training in gerontology or geriatrics. Policymakers will need to develop policies that train professionals and paraprofessionals to care for the aging population, and continue to recruit, retain, and retrain, the existing paraprofessional and professional workers as they age.

In order to ensure that aging and long-term care services are a policy priority in California over the next decades, advocacy needs to be redefined. The constituency for advocacy is changing. Although significant in their proportion relative to the overall population, baby boomers are increasingly diverse. In comparison to previous generations of older adults, baby boomers are better educated, more interested in personal choice and control, and more skeptical of government. The needs of vulnerable older adults are not disappearing but advocates also must acknowledge that not all older adults are vulnerable, nor are they united on any given prescription for social reform. In order for advocacy to remain relevant and responsive, the strategies must reflect this reality.

Advocacy for aging will require the development and continued support of coalitions across a range of stakeholders. Advocacy for older adults must incorporate a broader view. Other groups have needs just as pressing as those of older adults, and any advocacy strategy should be placed in the context of the entire community. Crosscutting issues, such as health insurance coverage for all Americans, and caregiving for those in need, can provide a forum on which aging advocates can collaborate with others, rather than competing for resources. By changing the advocacy framework to one that encompasses the needs of the entire community and places an emphasis on independence, flexibility, and choice, advocates will be more successful in their efforts.

In addition, California must develop a new pool of advocates. Increasing the pool of advocates and overall effectiveness of advocacy efforts in California will require a multilateral approach. Existing advocacy organizations and others within the aging network can be tapped for advocacy training and recruitment. Area Agency on Aging Advisory Councils are charged with advocacy through the federal Older Americans Act, but their effectiveness varies statewide. The California Commission on Aging is defined in California statute as the principle advocacy body for older Californians, yet their power and presence is not always visible. Advocates for older Californians aren't able to generate the groundswell of grassroots activity that other advocacy groups, such as those for children, people with disabilities, or the environment, are able to produce. All advocacy organizations for older Californians should look to other groups that have had success and adapt the best practices and proven methods to increase the voice of older Californians in shaping state policy.

Aging baby boomers will impact every area of state and local policy development. Since most of the major aging policy issues that need to be addressed are interrelated, policymakers, planners, and advocates can no longer continue to view and address specific topics and concerns independently. California's sheer size, diversity, and large older adult population make it a barometer of how the nation will grapple with the challenges and opportunities of population aging. California must begin reevaluating the adequacy of current policies and services to meet the needs of the state's aging population, especially in light of increasing diversity.[2]

Ensuring access to health care is essential for reducing mortality and disability and improving quality of life for all aging Californians, especially the oldest old. Overall differences in risks of disease, disability, and death in California's aging population are due to differences in health behaviors and environmental exposure, as well as access to health care and rehabilitation services. Policymakers can help decrease health problems by promoting preventive health programs, increasing geriatric training, and learning more about the changing health status of older adults[3]. Ultimately, the standard for health care will not only relate to physical health, but also the holistic health of the person – including physical and mental health and wellness.

A significant percentage of older Californians face serious housing-related problems. Many people over age 65, burdened with high housing costs and living on fixed incomes are in need of affordable housing. As baby boomers age, more will seek ways to remain independent at home and in the community, pressing for policies that create and replicate new models of elderly housing options that integrate housing and supportive services, including access to home modifications and the expansion of Universal Design. Universal Design is the design of products and environments to be useable by all people, to the greatest extent possible, without the need for adaptation or specialized design. Universal Design fits all users regardless of age, height, skill, or physical ability.

- Develop tax credits or deductions for home modifications.

- Ensure that local general plans include housing elements that adhere to California's Olmstead Plan by providing an adequate supply of home and community-based options for older adults and adults with disabilities.

- Develop continuing education modules and requirements for professionals such as contractors, occupational therapists, and others regarding home modifications.

- Strengthen the Multipurpose Senior Services Program (MSSP) provisions for home modifications by ensuring that local programs allocate sufficient funds for programs.

---

[2] Scharlach, Torres-Gil, & Kaskie (2001). *Strategic planning framework for an aging population.* California Policy Research Center, University of California.
[3] Satariano, W.A.; Villa, V. (2001). *The health status of older Californians.* California Policy Research Center, University of California.

⁑ Direct a percentage of local redevelopment funds **and the expansion of** for home modifications.

Mobility is critical to the well-being of California's elderly and persons with disabilities. To live full lives and avoid social isolation, people must be able to access friends and relatives, health care services, shopping opportunities, and social and recreational activities. Given that transportation needs are directly related to land-use planning, alternative transportation services, driver safety education, "walkable" communities, and better access to public transportation need to be fully developed throughout California.

In general, aging baby boomers have not prepared financially for their long futures. To prepare for the impending growth in California's aging population, government policies will need to provide incentives for employers and for workers to encourage individuals to remain in the work force. Policies will need to support individuals' continuance in the labor force for as long as they need or want to work.

Aging baby boomers will seek ways to increase volunteerism at all life stages as a way to stay productive and connected to society. A social model is needed through which aging baby boomers can optimize their continued involvement.

In recent decades, there has been a growing appreciation for the fact that older age, while a time of greater risk for declines in health and functioning, need not inevitably be associated with such negative outcomes. Health promotion activities consisting of exercise, nutritional guidance, and regular preventive physician visits will need to be greatly expanded if they are to have any meaningful and long-term positive impact upon both health maintenance and cost containment of health care expenditures. Many prevention programs will require an upfront investment of funds in order to produce long-term savings.

Family caregiving patterns are as varied as California's families – there is no "right way" of providing care that works for everyone[4]. Caregiving in California ranges from informal assistance provided by family members to skilled nursing services provided by certified professionals and paraprofessionals. Regardless of the setting, California faces a shortage among caregivers necessary to accommodate an aging population.

The availability of family caregivers to provide care is a major factor in predicting whether or not older people can remain at home. Approximately 75 percent of communitydwelling disabled elderly are cared for at home or in the community by family members or other

---

[4] Scharlach, A. (2001). *Family caregiving for older Californians*. California Policy Research Center, University of California.

informal care providers. **By 2007, an estimated four million Californians will be caregivers.** If California's family caregivers were paid $8 an hour, the typical wage of a home health aide, the cost of caregiving would be $22.1 billion a year. However, in most cases family members are not paid, and in fact' bear close to 40 percent of long-term care costs.

The aging baby boomers are changing the characteristics of the typical family unit; this will likely impact the needs and characteristics of caregiving in the future. Policymakers will need to develop systems that respond to the changing needs of caregivers, especially in such a mobile society.

Develop a single-payer universal health care system.

- Change health insurance practices to provide multi-year policies that include incentives to invest in prevention and reduce administrative costs.

- Establish tax credits for health insurance for those under the age of 65 – primarily targeting those between the ages of 55 and 65.

- Establish tax credits for individuals to purchase long-term care insurance at the state level.

- Increase federal and state funding for educating providers and older adults   regarding Medicare funds and relevant changes in Medicare coverage, especially for dual eligibles.

- Increase training among physicians and health care providers regarding palliative care.

- Invest in medication management technology and innovative programs for disease prevention and chronic disease management replicating best practices and pilot projects from other states.

- Expand the current Preventive Health Care for the Aging program statewide.

- Establish, develop, and fund statewide chronic disease self-management programs, particularly for heart disease and diabetes.

- Encourage the development of telemedicine and telehealth in rural communities, including the adjustment of reimbursement rate methodology.

- Adopt building codes that ensure that care facilities have the wiring and infrastructure needed to allow access to medical, telecommunications, and other technology at the time they are built to avoid costly retrofitting.

Aging baby boomers will prefer to receive their care at home and in the community, leading to the need for policies and funding streams that promote non-institutional caregiving and creative community-based long-term support arrangements. Existing funding for home and community-based services is not sufficient to meet the current demand, a demand that will only increase as the population ages[5].

Financial abuse is expected to be one of the most prevalent crimes committed against older adults. Policymakers will need to decrease aging baby boomers' susceptibility to scams and neglect. They should consider developing a method to prevent, prosecute, and punish those who commit financial crimes against older Californians' individual assets, pension, and retirement programs.

In order to promote wellness and inclusion of aging baby boomers in society, it will be important to change the way aging is perceived and to popularize more realistic images of what it means to be "old" – to expect positive experiences in later life. Policymakers will need to consider how to provide aging baby boomers with genuine choices about how they age.

Baby boomers are already changing the way that society views old age. They want more information, and they want more choices. They are struggling with the challenges of caring for their aging parents, raising their own children and grandchildren, and working towards their own retirement. The issues confronting aging are everywhere and intertwined with every aspect of our lives. It is precisely this interwoven tapestry of needs that demands a unified approach. Few of California's challenges will respond to a "one-size-fits-all" approach to policy development. The increasing diversity of the aging population demands creative solutions that take into account racial, ethnic, and cultural differences, as well as regional variations, and socioeconomic disparities[6].

California has never seen anything like the aging boom. No state has. There is no triedand true way to deal with something that has not happened before. We must draw the map ourselves. And we must realize that this map has to include every highway, every boulevard, every avenue, and alley. **Other states will watch how California grapples with its age wave. We will set the trends and establish the precedents, good or bad.** While California ages over the next several decades, there will be multiple opportunities for innovation and coordination. However, along with these opportunities for growth and change, there will be the

---

[5] Harrington, C.; Newcomer, R.; & Fox, P. (2001). *Long-term care for older Californians*. California Policy Research Center, University of California.

[6] Scharlach, Torres-Gil, & Kaskie (2001). *Strategic planning framework for an aging population*. California Policy Research Center, University of California.

temptation to maintain the status quo. All Californians will have to decide what type of future they want for their grandparents, parents, and themselves as they age.

To date, several of California's legislators have attempted, with varying degrees of success, to address many of the problems noted in this report. In many cases, successful legislation has taken years to develop, much to the frustration of policymakers, advocates, and consumers alike. California has made significant strides in elder abuse protection and increasing options for long-term care. Yet, in other cases, success has yet to materialize. Efforts to reorganize home and community-based programs at the state level, long-term care integration, universal health care, and replication of Oregon's Death with Dignity Act have made incremental progress over the last ten years but have not become law.

While policymakers can take the lead in addressing the challenges posed by the aging population, success is not possible without the support of advocates, service providers, scholars, and consumers themselves. This report is only the first step in developing solutions to the problems that California faces. With leadership and shared vision, the state can move bravely into a future in which older adults and adults with disabilities live longer, healthier, and more dignified lives, and do so in their own homes. We can lead the nation in demonstrating that resources can be managed wisely, and effectively, and that long-term investments make longterm rewards.

Changes in legislative and policy direction should include a benchmark or tool to determine what constitutes good and effective policy. Legislative and policy changes included in this report, as well as other legislation regarding older Californians, should meet the following three criteria:

In order to ensure that aging and long-term care services are a policy priority in California over the next decades, advocacy needs to be redefined. The constituency for advocacy is changing. Although significant in their proportion relative to the overall population, baby boomers are increasingly diverse. In comparison to previous generations of older adults, baby boomers are better educated, more interested in personal choice and control, and more skeptical of government. The needs of vulnerable older adults are not disappearing, but advocates also must acknowledge that not all older adults are vulnerable, nor are they united on any given prescription for social reform. In order for advocacy to remain relevant and responsive, the strategies must reflect this reality.

Advocacy for aging will require the development and continued support of coalitions across a range of stakeholders. Advocacy for older adults must incorporate a broader view. Other groups have needs just as pressing as those of older adults, and any advocacy strategy should be placed in the context of the entire community. Crosscutting issues, such as health insurance coverage for all Americans, and caregiving for those in need, can provide a forum on which aging advocates can collaborate with others, rather than competing for resources. By changing the advocacy framework to one that encompasses the needs of the entire community and places an emphasis on independence, flexibility, and choice, advocates will be more successful in their efforts.

In addition, California must develop a new pool of advocates. Increasing the pool of advocates and overall effectiveness of advocacy efforts in California will require a multi-lateral approach. Existing advocacy organizations and others within the aging network can be tapped for advocacy training and recruitment. Area Agency on Aging Advisory Councils are charged with advocacy through the federal Older Americans Act, but their effectiveness varies statewide. The California Commission on Aging is defined in California statute as the principle advocacy body for older Californians, yet their power and presence is not always visible. Advocates for older Californians aren't able to generate the groundswell of grassroots activity that other advocacy groups, such as those for children, people with disabilities, or the environment, are able to produce. All advocacy organizations for older Californians should look to other groups that have had success and adapt the best practices and proven methods to increase the voice of older Californians in shaping state policy.

Develop new models for training and recruiting advocates based on approaches from the Oklahoma Leadership Academy and the Senior Action Network in San Francisco. Build coalitions among a variety of advocacy groups to focus on common issues such as affordable housing and health care.

All Offer incentives and credits to builders to construct and remodel special needs and age-friendly housing near fixed transportation lines. Develop a statewide Housing Trust Fund for California for funding affordable housing seniors replicating other state models.

Mobility is critical to the well-being of California's elderly and persons with disabilities. To live full lives and avoid social isolation, people must be able to access friends and relatives, health care services, shopping opportunities, and social and recreational activities. Given that transportation needs are directly related to land-use planning, alternative transportation services, driver safety education, "walkable" communities, and better access to public transportation need to be fully developed throughout California.

Provide for the development of Mobility Management Centers and include service coordination requirements. The Mobility Management Centers could serve to inventory volunteer transportation providers, direct clients to services, and minimize duplication and overlap among providers to maximize resources through service coordination. Define the mission of consolidated transportation service agencies in statute and identify resources with which they can fulfill their mission to become mobility managers.

Ensure that regional and local bicycle and pedestrian planning efforts consider and fund projects to make paths to fixed-route transit services accessible and usable by older pedestrians and those using mobility aides. Require that all local transit system plans address older adults and persons with disabilities, and require Area Agencies on Aging, Independent Living Centers, and others to coordinate with local public transportation planners when developing strategic plans. Even Improve access to routine physical and behavioral health care and health-related screenings with the use of mobile health clinics and temporary health clinics at locations where older adults congregate.

Develop and authorize the use of advance directives for mental health care replicating models in other states, such as Washington. Amend the intent language of the Older Californians Act to specifically address the issue of isolation and its consequences among older adults. Establish and/or expand mental health hotlines, linking them with Area Agency on Aging Information and Assistance providers. Develop statewide alcohol and substance abuse prevention and treatment programs targeted to the special needs of older adults. Develop statewide depression and suicide prevention programs tailored to the special needs of older adults.

Expand Gatekeeper models and programs for mental health. Gatekeeper models work with first responders and community members to educate them on strategies for identifying, interacting, and making referrals for older adults and people with disabilities who may be living with mental health issues. Develop training and continuing education programs for mental health professionals to ensure that they acquire expertise in the assessment, treatment, and appropriate referral of older adults with mental illness.

Financial abuse is expected to be one of the most prevalent crimes committed against older adults. Policymakers will need to decrease aging baby boomers' susceptibility to scams and neglect. They should consider developing a method to prevent, prosecute, and punish those who commit financial crimes against older Californians' individual assets, pension, and retirement programs.

Work with financial institutions to develop educational tools and prevention programs. Develop oversight protocols for financial institution employees who manage trusts. Ensure that the conservatorship system prevents abuse through the licensure of conservators, restrictions on the sale of property, and increased oversight.

Increase the enforcement of current elder and dependent adult abuse laws, including fraud prevention. Increase prosecution and fines for those who participate in brokerage scams involving inappropriate insurance and securities investments. Increase penalties and fines for false advertising and bait and switch tactics related to the sale of annuities.

Provide tax incentives to promote the development of active community environments, home technology, and accessibility. Develop incentives for developers to incorporate Universal Design features into single and multi- family housing, including fee reductions and tax incentives. Create a certification program for developers and architects that they can use to advertise their Universal Design compliance. Adopt a mandatory, cost-neutral, Universal Design standard for all new construction and major remodeling projects using state funds. Integrate Universal Design features and standards into local systems for awarding bids to publicly-financed housing.

Expand upon the existing Medicaid 1915 (c) waiver for assisted living pilot projects, and fully establish assisted living as a Medi-Cal benefit. Encourage the federal government to provide tax credits or other incentives for HUD Section 202 housing with service coordination components. Maintain and expand low-income tax credits and other financial supports to provide equity in new and existing developments. Increase the 10 percent reserve for preservation within the Low-Income Housing Tax Credit. Require the California Housing Finance Agency to provide incentives for senior housing development applicants to link housing with services and award more points in the competitive ranking process to housing developments that demonstrate innovation in service delivery through partnerships with service providers and other organizations.

Dixon Arnett (Chair): Professor/Lecturer, Gerontology, San Diego State University; Former Director, California Department of Aging; Former Assemblymember

Pauline Abbott: Professor, Gerontology, California State University, Fullerton

Joaquin Anguera: Professor, Gerontology, San Diego State University; Former Chief Deputy Director, San Diego Area Agency on Aging

Dion Aroner: Lobbyist; Former Assemblymember

Patty Berg: Assemblywoman; Chair, Assembly Committee on Aging & Long-Term Care

Ann Burns Johnson: Executive Director, California Association of Homes and Services for the Aging

Ronald Lee: Professor, Demography and Economics; Director, Center on the Economics and Demography of Aging, University of California, Berkeley

Ray Mastalish: Executive Director, California Commission on Aging

Erin O'Keefe: Lobbyist

Tom Porter: State Director, California State AARP

Allison Ruff: Principal Consultant, Assembly Committee on Aging and Long-Term Care

Andrew Scharlach: Professor, Social Welfare; Director, Center for the Advance Study of Aging Services, University of California, Berkeley

Steve Schmoll: Executive Director, Council on Aging, Silicon Valley

Sarah S. Steenhausen: Consultant, Senate Subcommittee on Aging & Long-Term Care

Peter Spaulding: Executive Director, California Association of Coordinated Transportation

Fernando Torres-Gil: Professor, Social Welfare; Director, Center for Policy Research on Aging, University of California, Los Angeles; Former Assistant Secretary, Administration on Aging

*In July 2004, report contributors participated in a three-day conference to establish the legislative priorities included in this report.

B. Family and Elder Care in the Twenty-First Century

Families and Elder Care in the Twenty-First Century

Ann Bookman and Delia Kimbrel

Summary - Although most Americans know that the U.S. population is aging, they are far less informed about the reality of providing elders with personal care, health care, and social support. Families—particularly women—have always been critical in providing elder care, but the entry of so many women into the paid labor force has made elder care increasingly difficult. Ann Bookman and Delia Kimbrel show how changes in both work and family life are complicating families' efforts to care for elderly relatives. Because almost 60 percent of elder caregivers today are employed, many forms of caregiving must now be "outsourced" to nonfamily members. And because elders are widely diverse by race and socioeconomic status, their families attach differing cultural meanings to care and have widely different resources with which to accomplish their care goals. Although the poorest elders have access to some subsidized services, and the wealthiest can pay for services, many middle-class families cannot afford services that allow elders to age in their homes and avoid even more costly institutional care.

Six key groups—health care providers, nongovernmental community-based service providers, employers, government, families, and elders themselves—are engaged in elder care, but their efforts are often fragmented and uncoordinated. All six groups must be able to work in concert and to receive the resources they need. Both employer and government policies must be improved. Although large businesses have taken up the elder care challenge, most small and mid-sized firms still do not offer flexible work arrangements. Social Security and Medicare have provided critical support to families caring for elders, yet both face significant financial short-falls. The Older American Act and the National Family Caregiver Support Program have broadened access to elder services, but need updating to address the needs of today's employed caregivers and elders who want to "age in place." And just over half of the nation's workforce is eligible for the unpaid leave benefits provided by the Family and Medical Leave Act.

The authors close by reflecting on the need for a coordinated, cross-sector movement to create an **"aging-friendly" society in the United States—a society that values well-being across the life span and supports citizens from diverse cultures and income levels as they age.** www.futureofchildren.org Ann Bookman is a visiting scholar and senior lecturer, adjunct, and Delia Kimbrel is a doctoral candidate, at the Heller School for Social Policy and Management at Brandeis University.

For most of the nation's history, caring for the elderly was a family affair carried out largely by women in the home. As the twenty-first century unfolds, however, elder care in the United States is an increasingly complex enterprise, with much personal care "outsourced" to paid nonfamily caregivers. Today elder care is a multisector undertaking with six key stakeholder groups—health care providers, nongovernmental community-based service agencies, employers, government, families, and elders themselves. The six groups, however, often work separately, or even at cross-purposes. They must be better integrated and resourced to ensure that seniors can age with dignity, families can receive appropriate supports, and society can manage the costs associated with geriatric health care and elder economic security. In this article we examine the changing demographics of elders and families; what it means to engage in care work of an elderly parent or relative; how caregiving varies by race, gender, and socioeconomic status; and institutional responses to the challenges of caregiving from employers and the government. We close with reflections on the need for a coordinated, cross-sector movement to create an "agingfriendly" society in the United States—a society that values well- being across the life course and seeks multi- generational solutions.

Changing Demographics with the numbers of older Americans rapidly growing ever larger, the landscape of elder care in the United States is changing. During the past century, the population of Americans aged sixty-five and older increased eleven- fold.

1.	According to the 2010 census, 13 percent of the population, or 40.3 million individuals, were sixty-five or older.

2.	The population share of those aged eighty-five and older, sometimes called the "oldest old," was 1.1 percent. By 2030 approximately 80 million Americans, or 20 percent of the population, are projected to be sixty-five or older, and 2.3 percent of the population will be eighty-five and older.

3.	In addition to its increasing numbers over the coming decades, the elderly population will change in a variety of ways—more people will live longer and healthier lives, the number of older males will grow, and the group's racial and ethnic diversity will increase.

4.	But not all trends are positive. Although the poverty rate among the elderly fell from 25 percent in 1970 to 13 percent in 1992, as the real median income of both males and females increased,

5.	in 2009, approximately 12.9 per- cent of people 65 and older still had incomes at the poverty level.

6.	The Great Recession that began in 2007 eroded the economic status of moderateincome and middle-class elders, many of whom saw their pensions and 401(k)s decrease, the value of their homes decline, and their other financial investments lose value.

7.	Clearly these changes in the nation's elderly population will present challenges to family members who help provide elder care. And other national demographic shifts—delayed marriage and childbearing for young adults, decreased family size, and changes in family composition and structure—are complicating that challenge.

Increased longevity among elders not only extends the years of caregiving by their adult children but may require their grandchildren to become caregivers as well. Married couples may have as many as four elderly parents living; in fact, they may have more parents or relatives in need of care than they have children living at home VOL. 21 / NO. 2 / FALL 2011 119 Families and Elder Care in the Twenty-First Century or on their own. In the past, research on elder care focused on the challenges facing working adults who were caring for both children and elderly parents—the so-called sandwich generation—a term coined by sociologist Dorothy Miller to refer to specific generational inequalities in the exchange of resources and support.

8.	Miller's research highlighted the stress on the middle generation of employees who are caring for two groups of dependents while receiving little support. The sandwich metaphor, however, is outmoded in several respects: it does not convey that more than one generation may provide elder care or that members of any generational cohort can be both caregivers and care receivers. Nor does the image of static layers do justice to the dynamic interaction between generations, such as transfers of financial aid, sharing residential space, or exchanging personal and emotional care. Today researchers are increasingly finding that adults may spend more years caring for their parents than caring for their children.

9.	And because families today tend to be small, middle-aged adults may have smaller sibling networks to share elder care responsibilities. In short, elder care in the United

States is a demanding task, and caregivers, especially the almost 60 percent of family caregivers who are employed, are finding it harder to undertake that task alone.

10.   Care Work and the Dimensions of Elder Caregiving There is an extensive body of research on family "care work" dating back to the 1960s with a study that challenged the "myth of the abandoned elderly" and showed that families were still caring for elders, but that changes in external conditions in the family, the workplace, and the community were making caregiving more challenging.

11.   One of the contributions of recent care work research is to draw attention to the "work" aspects of caregiving. This framing contradicts personal and cultural ideas about why families care for elders and makes two related arguments: the first is that because family caregiving is largely done by women and is unpaid, it is often devalued; the second is that despite this devaluing, unpaid care work adds huge value to U.S. society in providing much needed care and "services" to the most vulnerable in the nation's population. Some scholars have tried to calculate the monetary value of unpaid care work to strengthen the argument about its value. Estimates vary from $196 billion a year, calculated in 1997,

12.   to $257 billion a year based on a subsequent study by the United Hospital Fund in 2004.

13.   In either case, the numbers far exceed what the United States spends on home health care and nursing home care, underscoring the importance of family care. To differentiate the work families provide from the work that professionals and paraprofessionals provide, many studies of caregiving use the terms "informal care" to refer to the care provided by families and "formal care" to refer to that provided by trained health and social service staff. The distinction creates a sharp line between the informal care that is unpaid and takes place in private homes and the formal care that is paid and takes place in institutional and community settings. The distinction, however, has been challenged by some elder care scholars who find that family caregivers of elders provide care in hospitals, rehabilitation facilities, outpatient clinics, and community agencies. Family caregivers are a "shadow workforce" in the geriatric health care system.

14.   Some states are piloting "cash and counseling" programs to pay families for the elder care they do, so the paid-unpaid distinction is being challenged in public policies. 120 THE FUTURE OF CHILDREN Ann Bookman and Delia Kimbrel Elder care entails a variety of supports and responsibilities, many of which can change in intensity and complexity over time. Cultural differences unique to elders and their families shape their views on what aging, health, and end of life mean and thus affect expectations about who provides care and what is provided.

15.   The variations in elder care are numerous, as the following eight dimensions illustrate. Time Dimension Elder care takes three forms: short-term, intermittent, and long-term. Elderly parents may, for example, have surgery that immobilizes them temporarily, but restores them to a high level of daily functioning. In such cases the care needed may be fairly intense but of short duration, and so it disrupts the care-giver's job, family, and personal life, but only temporarily. In contrast, the seven in ten care recipients who have chronic health conditions

16.   may require intermittent care that entails regular trips to one or more specialists, medication management, and adjustments to household and personal routines. In such cases, the caregiver is needed frequently over a longer period and may be hard pressed to integrate caregiving demands with paid work. In other cases, elder care may be long-term, lasting for months or years. Such caregiving may be required on a daily basis and can seriously complicate the caregiver's ability to maintain a job, provide care for other family members, and maintain

personal and com- munity involvement. Since 1987 the American Association of Retired Persons (now called AARP) and the National Alliance for Caregiving (NAC) have conducted several national surveys tracking the time Americans invest in elder care.

17.   The most recent survey, in 2009, found intermittent elder care to be the type most commonly provided. Caregivers surveyed in that poll report providing such care for an average of 4.6 years; 31 percent report giving such care for more than five years.

18.   Half of all of caregivers spend eight hours or less a week, while 12 percent spend more than forty hours. Short-term or intermittent care may evolve into long-term care as an elder's physical or mental function, or both, deteriorates. Geographic Dimension The distance between an elder's place of residence and that of the caregiver has a major effect on the type and frequency of care. Because some American families are mobile—about 16 percent of families move each year

19.—adult children sometimes live in different cities, states, or even regions from their elderly parents. According to the most recent AARP-NAC survey data, 23 percent of caregivers live with the elder for whom they are caring (co-residence is particularly common among lowincome caregivers) and 51 percent live twenty minutes away.

20.   Long-distance caregiving, however, has been on the rise over the past fifteen years.

21.   One study by MetLife finds that at least 5 million caregivers live an hour or more away from the elder for whom they care.

22.   Of this group, about 75 percent provide help with daily activities, such as shopping, transportation, and managing household finances. Most long-distance caregivers share responsibilities with siblings or paid caregivers, or both. Several studies document that adult children who live near an elderly relative are most likely to provide the majority of elder care,

23.   underscoring the importance of geographic location. Residential Dimension To move, or not to move? Many elders struggle with this question, and often turn to family caregivers for help with the answer. Most elders want to live in their own homes and neighborhoods; for some, safety and accessibility require home renovations. Family caregivers may plan, organize, and finance adaptations in an elder's living space. Not all elders and all caregivers are home- owners (some are renters), which can pose particular challenges for all parties.

24.   When it is not feasible for elders to adapt their dwelling, moving becomes necessary. In that case, caregivers often research, plan, and organize the move. Some elders move to continuing care retirement communities that provide different types of units for residents of different abilities.

25.   Although such communities have grown in popularity, and may relieve families of some responsibilities, the units are expensive to buy, and monthly maintenance fees are costly, thus making this option unaffordable for most elders. A small share of elders lives in rehabilitation facilities, usually on a short-term basis. Between 5 and 6 percent of elders live in a long-term-care facility or nursing home, with caregivers making regular or intermittent trips to visit and monitor the care being provided. Most elders live in their own homes,

26.   which must be constantly assessed for safety and the availability of community services such as transportation, social services, and recreational opportunities. Nongovernmental organizations (NGOs) help maintain more than 10 million elders a day with long-term care supports and services so they can continue to live in their homes independently.

27. To help caregivers assess what is required for independent living, researchers have developed tools that can aid in choosing appropriate housing and support services.

28. Financial Dimension The economic resources available to caregiving families vary widely. Upper-middle-class and affluent families usually have adequate funds to pay for elder care services, while poor families are usually eligible for a variety of subsidized services, such as home health care. The hardest-hit families are the working poor and those with moderate incomes, who are too "rich" to qualify for subsidized services but unable to pay for care themselves. Many families caring for elderly relatives encounter this type of "middle-class squeeze." Researchers who explore the financial dimension of elder care find that crossgenerational transfers are fairly common. In a 2005 study, 29 percent of baby boomers provided financial assistance to a parent in the previous year, while about a fifth received financial support from a parent.

29. A recent nationally representative survey of elders over sixty- five offers a slightly different picture: half of these elders say they have given money to their adult children, while about a third say they help their adult children with childcare, errands, housework, and home repairs. When asked what their adult children give them, more than 40 percent report receiving help with errands and rides to appointments; about a third, help with housework and home repairs; and about a fifth, help with bill paying and direct financial support.

30. What is striking is that care, time, and money are being exchanged between the generations, going both ways. Health Dimension Some caregivers provide help in a short-term acute health care crisis, others care for elders with one or more chronic diseases, and a third group cares for elders with long-term incurable or progressive diseases. Families are a critical resource for the nation's health care system when they care for a relative with a debilitating disease, such as dementia or Alzheimer's, for which paid care is very expensive. Giving such care, however, is a major burden on these families, who frequently find that caregiver training—both how to manage the behavior and symptoms of the elder and how to cope with their own feelings—is often not available.

31. The health status of an elder determines the extent of a caregiver's involvement with personal care, often referred to as activities of daily living, such as eating, bathing, toileting, and dressing, or as instrumental activities of daily living, such as cooking, shopping, and bill paying. The health status of the elder also shapes the extent of caregivers' involvement in medical tasks such as giving medications; dressing wounds after surgery; checking weight, blood pressure, and blood sugar levels; and monitoring medical equipment. A national survey of caregivers found that more than 40 percent helped with one or more medical tasks, even though only one- third reported that they had the training to do so.

32. That finding underscores the "medicalization" of the care work that families are providing for elders. One elderly cohort that is growing is "frail elders," defined as those sixtyfive and older who do not live in nursing homes but have difficulty with at least one aspect of independent living or are severely disabled, or both. This group numbered about 10.7 million people in 2002.

33. Analyses of a national data set showed that two-thirds of frail elders receive help—an average of 177 hours a month—with personal care from an unpaid family caregiver. More than half of that help comes from their daughters, most of whom are working.

34. Legal and Ethical Dimension When significant declines in physical and mental health compromise elders' ability to manage their own affairs, it is usually the family caregiver who assumes some level of control, decision-making power, and ultimately legal authority such

as power of attorney. Studies on the legal issues of elders often focus, particularly when financial resources are involved, on the caregiver as a source of interfamilial conflict and even elder abuse. A recent study of financial elder abuse, however, found that only 16.9 percent of the perpetrators were family members.

35.   Legal issues may also require caregivers to take on complex health-related roles, such as acting as health care proxy or setting up an advance directive or DNR (do not resuscitate) order. These steps can involve complex ethical questions and decisions, such as when to discontinue life supports for a terminally ill parent. Studies on elders at the end of life show the critical role that family caregivers play once palliative care is chosen, including assisting elders with daily living, handling medications, and making medical decisions.

36.   Using ethnographic data, a study of one elderly mother and her daughter documents how this family navigated the health care system and brought their own cultural meaning to endof-life care.

37.   Other studies emphasize the high degree of stress on families with terminally ill elders, showing VOL. 21 / NO. 2 / FALL 2011 123 Families and Elder Care in the TwentyFirst Century the unresponsiveness of some health care systems, as well as the ways in which community services can ease stress.

38.   Emotional, Moral, and Spiritual Dimension Much of the research on elder care explores the practical daily routines involved in personal care, health care, and housing. The emotional care that families provide, although essential to the well-being of elders, is less studied and is difficult to define. The medical anthropologist Arthur Kleinman, a caregiver for his wife with Alzheimer's, argues that the emotional part of caregiving is in essence a moral act—"an existential quality of what it is to be a human being."

39.   Attending to the spiritual needs of elders for whom religious experience, practice, and faith have been important is also critical to sustaining their physical and mental health and longevity.

40.   For these elders, caregivers' tasks include: spiritual and well-being assessments; using a reminiscence-and-life-review approach; identifying and facilitating contact with religious services, organizations, and clergy; and discussing end-of-life issues.

41.   Tailoring these tasks to an individual elder's particular faith tradition is both time-consuming and extremely meaningful. Outsourcing Elder Care and Care Coordination When family members cannot provide care, particularly if they are full-time workers or long-distance caregivers, or both, their job is to find an agency close to where the elder lives that will provide services for a fee. It takes time and effort to find an appropriate multiservice or aging service agency,

42.   to provide the agency with detailed personal and health information about the elder to ensure a good "client-provider fit," and to monitor services to be sure that needs are met and the elder is comfortable with the provider. Carrying out all these tasks to find just one type of service is difficult enough; if an elder needs multiple services, the work for the family can be significant. Many studies have documented the fragmentation in the geriatric health care and social services system, and others have called for greater care coordination to support caregivers.

43.   The handoffs between hospitals and families, or between rehabilitation facilities and families, can often be unsafe and unsatisfying, and the need for improved communication is widely documented.

44.   Given the cross-institutional complexities, some caregivers hire a geriatric care manager—often a trained social worker—to identify, monitor, and coordinate services. Hiring a

care manager requires research by the family caregiver, as well as ongoing monitoring and extensive communication. The work of care coordination is a significant, often unnoticed, aspect of care many families do themselves, either because they cannot afford to hire a geriatric care manager or because they prefer to keep an eye on things themselves.

45. Elder Caregiving and Diversity Most studies on aging and elder care treat elders and their caregivers as monolithic groups. But as the nation has become more diverse, so too has the population of elders. Elder caregiving varies by gender, race, and socioeconomic status, and families from African American, Latino, Asian, Native American, and other groups bring their own strengths and needs to the caregiving experience. Although gender, race, and socioeconomic status are treated separately below, it is important to note that these variables often intersect in powerful and important ways in the lives of caregivers. An "intersectionality" approach shows how unequal opportunity over the life course shapes trajectories of advantage and disadvantage for elders and the families who care for them. Future research must explore multiple aspects of diversity in order to develop new policies that address the interaction between socio- economic inequality and differences based on gender, race, and culture. Gender and Elder Care Elderly women live longer than do elderly men, and despite a lifetime of providing care to others, they are more likely than men to live alone, live in poverty, and lack care themselves when they are elderly.

46. Research on gender and caregiving has two major themes. First, the majority (67 percent) of family caregivers are women,

47. with wives providing care to spouses and adult daughters providing the majority of care to elderly parents. Second, given the persistence of gender inequality in the workforce, including the gender gap in wages, women caregivers are more likely than men to cut back on work hours or quit their jobs because of their caregiving duties and are thus left with less income, small savings, and reduced pensions. Although women in the general population have greater elder care responsibilities than do men, recent studies reveal that employed women and employed men provide care in roughly equal numbers.

48. But gender differences persist nonetheless: employed women are more likely than employed men to provide family care on a regular basis, they spend more hours providing care, and they spend more time providing direct care such as meal preparation, household work, physical care, and transportation.

49. This finding is consistent with other evidence on gender trends in elder care showing that women tend to perform household and personal care tasks that are physically draining and likely to interrupt daily activities, while men tend to give periodic assistance.

50. Both working and nonworking male caregivers receive more assistance with their caregiving efforts than do women; they also tend to delegate their tasks to others and to seek paid assistance to alleviate some of their caregiving responsibilities.

51. Despite the growing number of men balancing work and elder care responsibilities, women are particularly vulnerable to negative work-related consequences.

52. Women who are caring for elders generally reduce their work hours, leave the workforce, or make other adjustments that have negative financial or career implications. Some refuse overtime and pass up promotions, training, assignments that are more lucrative, jobs requiring travel, and other challenging but time-consuming job opportunities.

53. Many low-income women and women of color who are employed do not have sufficient flexibility or autonomy in their jobs to be able to take an elderly parent to the doctor or attend to other needs.

54.   Despite feelings of satisfaction from their care, caregivers can sometimes feel burdened, socially isolated, strained, and hopeless. A recent MetLife study of working caregivers, based on a large corporate employer's health risk appraisal database of roughly 17,000 respondents, found that employed women are significantly more likely than employed men caregivers to self-report negative effects on personal well-being.

55.   Caregivers in general report more physical and mental health problems than noncaregivers,

56.   and more female caregivers (58 per- cent) report negative health effects than male caregivers (42 percent).

57.   In a study assessing gender differences in caregiver health, VOL. 21 / NO. 2 / FALL 2011 125 Families and Elder Care in the Twenty-First Century Martin Pinquart and Silvia Sörenson found that women had lower scores for subjective well-being and perceived physical health, as well as higher scores for burden and depression than men. The effects for women care- givers indicated a positive and statistically significant relationship.

58.   Race, Ethnicity, and Elder Care The growing diversity of the United States makes it important for researchers to con- sider how race and ethnicity—both socially constructed categories—shape aging and the caregiving experience. The nation's legacy of racial oppression and structural inequality has created socioeconomic inequities in education, health, housing, income, and wealth. Many low-income men and women of color enter old age after a lifetime of cumulative disadvantage, during which limited access to economic opportunity has obstructed efforts to accumulate savings for retirement and limited access to health care has led to poorer health. Few families from racial and ethnic minority groups use paid or outsourced care, and those who do can sometimes face structural barriers in accessing them. Although most Americans refrain from putting their elderly kin in nursing homes, Latinos, African Americans, and Asians are least likely to do so.

59.   Even elders of color with greater care needs, such as those afflicted with dementia or chronic illnesses, are more likely than whites to receive care from their children and live in the community with them.

60.   Many studies show that families of color rely on extended kin networks and friends for financial assistance, material goods, domes- tic duties, and other supports.

61.   African Americans, especially, rely on networks of neighbors, friends, and fellow congregants. Language and cultural barriers often lead Chinese American and Puerto Rican caregivers to use ethnically oriented organizations in their communities for support.

62.   Extensive social support may partially explain why racial and ethnic minority groups tend to have more favorable attitudes toward caregiving and higher caregiving satisfaction.

63.   Studies suggest that many groups of color value mutual exchange, reciprocity, filial responsibility, and interdependence, whereas Western European and white ethnic groups value self-reliance and independence. Using well-established positive appraisal scales and coping questionnaires, several studies find a significant "race" effect, with caregivers of color such as African Americans and Latinos showing the highest appraisals of positive aspects of caregiving and higher scores on well-being measures.

64.   Among some Latino groups, the extended family is expected to provide care to older relatives,

65.   and Native Americans strongly value giving back to those who have provided for them, reinforcing the value of reciprocity in their culture.

66.   White caregivers report greater depression and view caregiving as more stressful than do caregivers of color.

67.   Studies that have addressed racial and ethnic growing diversity of the United States makes it important for researchers to consider how race and ethnicity shape aging and the caregiving experience. Differences among caregivers generally have not focused on working caregivers. One that does finds that employed white caregivers report significantly higher work demand and strain than Latino and black working caregivers.

68.   Although research consistently reveals significant differences in caregiver outcomes by race, findings may vary because of differences in recruitment strategies, in criteria for inclusion and exclusion, in construct measurement, in research instruments, and in statistical techniques. The studies also vary in sample size and sampling strategy and rarely use random assignment or national probability sampling to posit any causal relationships between variables. To strengthen generalizability, accuracy of statistical findings, and comparability across studies, researchers will have to use more diverse and random sampling strategies as well as experimental and mixed qualitative and quantitative methodologies.

69.   Socioeconomic Status and Elder Care Although researchers do not often explore the implications of socioeconomic status— defined by education, occupational status, family income, net worth, and financial assets—for elder care, it can nevertheless have important effects on elders' quality of life and the kind of care their families can provide. In the first place, many low-income elders have insufficient resources. More than half of all senior households (54 percent) cannot meet their expenses even using their combined financial net worth, Social Security benefits, and pension incomes.

70.   Among older persons reporting income in 2008, 20.3 percent had less than $10,000.

71.   Such eco- nomic challenges often increase the financial burden, hardship, and strain on their families. Many studies do show that families with higher socioeconomic status tend not to provide physical care themselves, and instead tend to purchase elder care services, provide financial gifts, buy alternative lodging, and remodel homes to accommodate an elder.

72.   A scarcity of resources makes working poor and working-class caregivers more likely to provide direct care themselves rather than to hire professional care managers. When low- income families do purchase formal services, they use them only for short periods. Middle-class and higher-income caregivers hire elder care assistance for longer periods or until their resources run out.

73.   Responses from Employers and Government Researchers have also investigated how employers and government are responding to the challenges families face in providing elder care. Are employers, for example, providing working caregivers of elders with "family- friendly" benefits and policies? Are federal, state, and local governments meeting the needs of elders and caregivers with public policies? We explore the adequacy of their responses to the needs of both elders and family caregivers to gain insight into what policy changes may be needed in the future. Responses from Employers Given the aging of the population and the high rate of female labor force participation, the share of elder caregivers who are employed has been growing over the past thirty years and is expected to continue, nearing the percentage of employees with childcare responsibilities. One of the earliest national estimates, based on data from the 1982 National Long-Term Care Survey and its companion National Informal Caregivers VOL. 21 / NO. 2 /

Families and Elder Care in the Twenty-First Century Survey, was that 15.8 percent of elder caregivers were employed,

74.	9 percent had quit their jobs because of elder care responsibilities, and 20 percent were experiencing conflict between work and elder care.

75.	Surveys conducted in the late 1980s and 1990s found the share of employed caregivers rising significantly, up to 64 percent in 1997.

76.	One 2010 study found that six in ten family caregivers are employed.

77.	another found that considered as a group, 50 percent of employed caregivers of elders work full time, and 11 percent work part time. In the coming years, employers will need to respond to the elder care needs of their workforce lest they compromise the performance of their firms and the retention of some of their most valued employees. Research on work and family conflict is extensive, and many studies focus on work and elder care for employees.

78.	Beyond general feelings of role conflict, working caregivers in one study report using their own sick leave or vacation hours to accommodate elder care needs (48 percent), cutting back on hours or quitting their job (37 percent), taking an additional job or increasing their hours to get funds for elder care expenses (17 percent), taking unpaid leave (15 percent), and leaving their job for a different one (14 percent).

79.	Many studies report negative health consequences for employed caregivers, including increased risk of stress and depression, diabetes, hypertension, and even premature death.

80.	If caregivers cut back work hours, take unpaid leaves, or leave their jobs, the negative effects can go beyond the individual caregivers themselves to include whole families. For example, a MetLife study documented negative financial repercussions for families from shortterm income losses, long-term losses of retirement savings, and lost opportunities for career advancement.

81.	Researchers are also examining the policies and programs of employers to address their employees' elder care needs; rough estimates are that from 25 to 50 percent of employers offer these programs.

82.	Large firms are more likely than small companies to have elder care programs, and a
2003 study estimates that 50 percent of large corporations offer such programs.

83.	For small and mid-sized firms, the estimate was 26 percent in 2006 and 22 percent in 2007.

84.	Studies on how the recent recession affected elder care programs are just now becoming available; one, for example, shows that most employers are maintaining workplace flexibility, although reduction of hours may translate into reduction in pay, so increased flexibility entails both costs and benefits.

85.	Elder Care Assistance Programs, introduced by companies during the late 1980s, have grown in scope. The early programs— paralleling those developed to support workers with young children—included resource and referral services to locate elder care services in the elder's community, and flexible spending accounts for putting aside funds on a pre-tax basis to cover elder care expenses.

86.	During the 1990s, some companies expanded elder care benefits through Employee Assistance Programs or new "work-life programs" to include flexible work arrangements (58 percent), personal or sick leaves (16 percent), and access to short-term emergency backup care when a paid care- giver was unexpectedly absent (4 percent).

87.   During the mid-1990s, some researchers began exploring the question of whether employees made use of elder care benefits. Early studies found that use rates were low, although the range was fairly-wide—from 2 to 34 percent—with use by employees in private-sector firms lower than use by public-sector employees.

88.   Most scholars and human resource managers hypothesize that rates were low because employers had not publicized the programs that were available. A 2007 survey of human resource managers at Fortune 500 companies found that flexible work arrangements and leave programs were the most highly utilized and had the best use-to-cost ratio.

89.   Emergency short- term home care had the lowest use rates and highest cost, and thus the worst use-to-cost ratio. In open-ended questions, respondents focused on the need for better communication about elder care programs; the importance of supervisors actively encouraging the use of these programs; and the difficulty of countering negative perceptions about these programs.

90.   Although elder care benefits appear to boost employee recruitment and retention, that link has not been conclusively demonstrated.

91.   To date, the needs of employed elder caregivers far exceed the employer response, and elder care assistance tends to be offered only by the largest employers. Some studies about "family-responsive" workplaces do not even mention elder care as a benefit needed by families,

92.   and the findings of studies that do focus on elder care have less than encouraging findings. The 2009 Age and Generations study found that employees who are caring for elders had less access to flexible work arrangements than did employees who were caring for their children or who had no dependent care responsibilities, that employees in the sandwich generation were less likely to be included in new projects based on teamwork than workers with no elder care demands,

93.   and that employees who provide elder care had lower job security than other groups.

94.   Elder care programs are still less frequently offered than childcare programs, and a 2006 study found that although almost three-quarters of employers offered some childcare assistance, only one-third offered elder care assistance.

95.   What accounts for employers' lag in offering elder care assistance? And how can work- places make elder care a key component of the work-family or work-life agenda? Elder care may have received less attention than childcare because ageism and denial about aging is deeply entrenched in U.S. culture. As Muriel Gillick, a palliative care physician, argues, "Contemporary Americans are eager to prevent, obliterate, or at least conceal old age...in keeping with the belief that we can control our destiny."

96.   This denial can lead employers to ignore or minimize the elder care needs of their workforce, using arguments about high costs and low utilization to justify having few elder care programs. Some work-family scholars argue that developing a family-friendly workplace is a long-term process with three distinct stages. In the first stage the goal is to promote the recognition of a particular work-family issue as a visible, legitimate need. In the second stage the goal is to implement and then refine specific programs, including effective communication and supervisor training. The third stage involves institutionalizing the new work-family programs into the culture of the workplace to heighten program reach and effectiveness.

97.   In this evolutionary paradigm, different percentages of companies are at different stages in responding to elder care. Many private-sector firms and the majority of small and midsized firms are still in the first stage, struggling to recognize elder care programs as a legitimate need of the work- force. Roughly a third of firms are in the second stage, starting, developing, and retaining elder care programs. Only a minority of firms—mainly large companies—are in the third stage. Making the "family-friendly workplace" an "elder-care-friendly work- place" remains an unrealized project for many employers. Responses from Government During the nineteenth and twentieth centuries the United States gradually transferred responsibility for elder care from the family to the government, from the private sphere to the public sphere.

98.   But despite landmark twentieth-century legislation, it can be argued that the United States lacks the full range of public policies needed to address the aging of the population, and that families still bear the primary responsibility. Table 1 briefly summarizes six public policies that are key to the well-being of elders and their family caregivers. Some have enhanced health and income security for elders; others have enhanced the supports available to both employed and non-employed family caregivers. We briefly address the strengths and weaknesses of some of these policies to suggest possible areas for policy expansion.

Social Security is critical to providing a basic level of financial support and security to elders. Several issues, however, weaken its effectiveness. Initially the system strength- ened intergenerational ties because those who retired—only 5.2 percent of the population Name of policy Year started Basic goal Eligibility Source of funds Social Security Act 1935 Provide income for people who have retired from paid employment Work in a Social Security- covered job for 10 years or more, can start collecting at age 62 up to age 70, widow(er)s at 60, disabled at 50 Payroll taxes and self- employment contributions, paid into Social Security Trust Fund by employees and employers Medicare 1965 Coverage of health care costs, including Part A: hospital care, Part B: outpatient care, and Part D: prescription drugs People 65 and older, who had Medicare-covered employment, not linked to income earned Employers and employees pay taxes for Part A, funds from SSI checks cover Part B, and Part D paid for by Medicare plus private insurance Medicaid 1965 Cover health care costs for low-income children and families, long-term care for elderly and/or disabled Pregnant women, children, teens, elders, blind, and disabled with low incomes Means-tested, funded by state and federal funds, managed by states Older Americans Act (OAA) 1965 Promote the delivery of social services to aging population via Administration on Aging (AoA) and state agencies National Elder Locator for all families, some meal programs, housing, and services for low-income elders Taxes and other government funds, most funding for social service programs, rest goes to jobs program, research, and training Family and Medical Leave Act 1993 Twelve weeks of job- protected unpaid leave with continuation of health benefits for own serious health condition, and/or care of seriously ill parent, child or spouse, and child rearing Workers at firms with 50 or more employees within 75-mile radius, who worked 1,250 hours and 12 consecutive months Payroll tax in California and New Jersey, otherwise unpaid Administrative costs funded by states and U.S. Department of Labor National Family Caregiver Support Program 2000, under OAA reauthorization Referrals for services/ respite care, information, counseling, training, and support groups for family caregivers Persons of any age who serve as unpaid caregivers for persons 60 years or older Funds from Older Americans Act, Title III E Table 1.

Institutional Responses to Aging and Elder Care from Government was sixty-five or older in 1930—were reaping benefits based on the productivity of younger workers. But in the decades ahead, more people will be needing retirement income, and fewer young workers will be available to replenish Social Security funds, thus putting pressure on the younger generation and creating tension between generations.

99. In addition, because Social Security is based on wages in the paid labor force, women who delayed work, interrupted work, or never entered the workforce because of family caregiving responsibilities have smaller benefits in old age than men (though at the death of her spouse, a woman is eligible to collect a "survivor" Social Security benefit). Medicare, a second foundational piece of economic security for elders, ensures coverage of many health care costs. It, too, how- ever, is problematic. Originally enacted to cover the costs of acute care and hospitalization, Medicare does not provide adequate insurance for chronic illnesses, those common to most elders. Medicare does not reimburse hospitals fully for the care they provide, so many hospitals have shortened patient stays, creating difficulties for caregivers when an elder is prematurely discharged to rehab or to home. Medicare will cover a stay in a skilled nursing facility only if daily nursing or rehab services are needed and will cover ten hours a week of home care only if skilled nursing care is required. Finally, Medicare does not cover the cost of long-term care. Medicaid, the third key government policy, is the largest source of payment for nursing home care, and it will become increasingly important as the nation's population ages. In 2008, nearly 41 percent of the nation's nursing facility care was paid by Medicaid, averaging nearly $30,000 for each beneficiary.

100. In most states, Medicaid also pays for some long-term care services at home and in the community. Although eligibility varies from state to state, those elders who are eligible for Medicaid assistance must have limited assets and incomes below the poverty line. They also must contribute all or most of their available income toward the cost of their care. Many elderlies who enter nursing homes pay for their own care initially. Once their resources have been depleted, however, they are covered by Medicaid. According to a study by Brenda Spillman and Peter Kemper, 16 percent of Medicaid users began by paying their own way in long-term nursing facilities, exhausted their resources, and converted to Medicaid; 27 percent were covered by Medicaid when they were admitted to the nursing home.

101. Medicaid often provides supplemental services to fill gaps left by Medicare. The Centers for Medicare and Medicaid Services estimated that Medicaid provided some additional health coverage for 8.5 million Medicare beneficiaries in 2009.

102. In addition, Medicare and Medicaid jointly fund a model program called PACE (Program of All-Inclusive Care for the Elderly), in which an interdisciplinary team, consisting of professional and paraprofessional staff, assesses participants' needs, develops care plans, and delivers all services (including acute care services and nursing facility services when necessary), which are Despite their many provisions for elder support, Medicaid and Medicare leave significant gaps in coverage. (VOL. 21 / NO. 2 / FALL 2011 131 Families and Elder Care in the Twenty-First Century) integrated for a seamless provision of total care. The program is available to individuals fifty-five and older who are certified by the state as nursing home eligible and meet the income and assets requirements to qualify for Medicaid.

103. Despite their many provisions for elder support, Medicaid and Medicare leave significant gaps in coverage. The new Patient Protection and Affordable Care Act of 2010 should ease some of the burdens by expanding drugs covered by Medicare Part D, the prescription drug program, improving prevention benefits such as free annual wellness visits, and changing the cost of Medicare Advantage plans. Mechanisms to control or reduce Medicare spending may or may not benefit elders, and a new Medicare and Medicaid Innovations Center

holds promise of testing new payment and service delivery models that could benefit elders and their families.

A fourth important policy with implications for elder care is the Older Americans Act (OAA), passed as part of Lyndon Johnson's "Great Society" reforms and the first public policy to recognize the importance of community-based NGOs in the elder care system. Although the OAA signaled a significant effort to systematize and broaden access to elder services, studies evaluating its effectiveness have had mixed findings. For example, studies of home care programs have found that although providers have had some success in managing the daily practical needs of elders, they have been less successful in dealing with emergencies or significant health issues or levels of impairment.

104. Studies have shown that home care is more effective than inpatient care and reduces the length of hospital stays, but little data are available on how OAA programs affect measures of quality of life for elders or caregivers.105 A book on OAA's Long-Term Care Ombudsman Program summarizes a number of issues cited in studies of other OAA programs. These include: a misalignment of resources and goals, which compromises program effectiveness; a lack of coordination between OAA programs and resources, which diminishes program effectiveness; and a lack of elder or caregiver empowerment to take control of elders' health care or make positive programs more sustainable and cost-effective.

106.   The Family and Medical Leave Act (FMLA) is the only law that deals specifically with the challenges of working and providing elder care. A bipartisan commission that conducted two nationally representative random-sample surveys to study the impact of the FMLA on employers and employees reported to Congress in 1996 that the law was not the burden to business that some had anticipated.

107.   In terms of ease of administration and impact on productivity, profitability, and performance, the law was found either to have "no noticeable effect" or, in some cases, to produce cost savings. On the employee side, the FMLA was found to be a boon to families in their caregiving roles. Most leaves were short, and concerns that employees would abuse the law and use it for recreational time off proved unwarranted. In fact, some "leave-needers" did not take advantage of the law because they could not afford an unpaid leave. The surveys were repeated in 2000 with largely comparable results for employers and employees.

108.   The major complaint from the employer community was the difficulty of administering "intermittent leaves," although employees find that type of leave useful for chronic health problems. Between the 1995 and 2000 surveys there was a statistically significant increase in the use of FMLA for elder care.

109.   From a policy perspective, the FMLA is like a minimum labor standard. It provides valuable protections to workers but has limitations that hamper its effectiveness. Access to FMLA, for example, is restricted to about 55 percent of the workforce because of eligibility requirements for firms and employees. The definition of "family" is limited to parent, child, and spouse, depriving many elderly relatives such as grandparents or aunts and uncles, as well as those who are members of the lesbian, gay, bisexual, and transgendered (LGBT) community or who are not legally married, of cover- age. And because the leave provided is unpaid, it is difficult for low-income workers to use.

Recently two states, California, and New Jersey, passed laws to establish paid leave programs, and a new study of the California law yields useful information about the applicability of these models for other states.

110. These new state policies are contemporary examples of the historical research of sociologist Theda Skocpol, who showed that federal policy is often driven by demands from local citizen associations and the actions of state legislatures.

111. Finally, the National Family Caregiver Support Program (NFCSP) is the first federal law to acknowledge fully the needs of caregivers regardless of their employment status. Preliminary studies have shown that the program is expanding caregivers' access to elder care information and providing needs assessments, support groups, and stress reduction programs.

112. Although NFCSP offers many excellent services, such as respite care, counseling, and training for family caregivers, the funds available to deliver them are limited, particularly in the area of respite care.

113. As with many OAA programs, the goals of the statute are not matched by the resources needed for nongovernmental agencies to carry them out. Although the (VOL. 21 / NO. 2 / FALL 2011 133 Families and Elder Care in the Twenty-First Century) Public policies must move in a universal direction, like Social Security and Medicare, to help transform U.S. communities and make housing, transportation, and open space accessible to all elders. There is a pressing need to better integrate non-governmental organizations in the health care and social service sectors and to ensure they are culturally responsive. Employers must be encouraged to give employees in both professional and hourly jobs access to flexible work arrangements including part-time work, paid leave policies, paid sick days, and other "elder-friendly" workplace benefits. Overall, these groups must work together to create a culture in which aging is seen as a natural part of the life course and caregiving is seen as a multigenerational enterprise of great value to children, adults, elders, and society. Elders themselves and their family caregivers, as well as the public and private sectors, must build support for social investment in the next generation.

Today's children will be the workers, citizens, and family caregivers who will care for the growing U.S. elderly population tomorrow. Focusing on children's healthy development and education will build their capacity to provide supportive care for the elders of future generations.

Endnotes

1. Frank B. Hobbs, "Population Profile of the United States: The Elderly Population," U.S. Census Bureau (www.census.gov/population/www/pop-profile/elderpop.html).

2. Census 2000 Brief, C2KBR/01-12, U.S. Census Bureau (2001).

3. Jennifer Cheeseman Day, Population Projections of the United States by Age, Sex, Race, and Hispanic Origin: 1993–2050, Current Population Reports, P25-1104, U.S. Census

Bureau (1993); Administration on Aging, Table 12, "Older Population as a Percentage of the Total Population, 1900–2050" (www.aoa.gov/ aoaroot/aging_statistics/future_growth/future_growth.aspx#age).

4.   U.S. Census Bureau, "Age: 2000," Census 2000 Brief, October 2001 (www.census.gov/prod/2001pubs/ c2kbr01-12.pdf).

5.   Wan He and others, "Sixty-Five Plus in the United States," Current Population Reports, Special Studies, Series P23-209 (Washington: December 2005).

6.   U.S. Census Bureau, Current Population Survey, Annual Social and Economic Supplements (www.census. gov/hhes/www/poverty/histpov/hstpov5.xls); U.S. Census Bureau, Historical Poverty Tables, table C, "Poverty Rates for Elderly and Non-Elderly Adults, 1966–2009."

7.   The percentage of homeless adults fifty and older appears to be increasing, particularly in cities. M. William Sermons and Meghan Henry, "Demographics of Homelessness Series: The Rising Elderly Population," National Alliance to End Homelessness (April 2010).

8.   Dorothy A. Milller, "The 'Sandwich' Generation: Adult Children of the Aging," Social Work 26, no. 5 (September, 1981): 419–23.

9.   Leslie Foster Stebbins, Work and Family in America: A Reference Handbook (Santa Barbara, Calif.: ABC-CLIO, 2001), p. 40.

10.   National Alliance for Caregiving and AARP, Caregiving in the United States (Washington: 2009), p. 53.

11.   E. Shanas and G. F. Streib, eds., Social Structure and the Family: Generational Relations (Englewood Cliffs, N.J.: Prentice-Hall, 1965).

12.   Peter S. Arno, Carol Levine, and M. N. Memmott, "The Economic Value of Informal Caregiving," Health Affairs 18, no. 2 (1999): 182–88.

13.   Carol Levine, ed. Always on Call: When Illness Turns Families into Caregivers (Vanderbilt University Press, 2004), p. 5.

14.   Ann Bookman and Mona Harrington, "Family Caregivers: A Shadow Workforce in the Geriatric Health Care System?" Journal of Health Policy, Politics and Law 32, no. 6 (2007): 1026.

15.   Carol Levine and Thomas H. Murray, eds., The Cultures of Caregiving: Conflict and Common Ground among Families, Health Professionals and Policy Makers (Johns Hopkins University Press, 2004).

16.   Family Caregiving in the U.S.: Findings from a National Survey (Washington: National Alliance for Caregiving and the American Association of Retired Persons, 1997). VOL. 21 / NO. 2 / FALL 2011 135 Families and Elder Care in the Twenty-First Century

17.   Donna Wagner, Comparative Analysis of Caregiver Data for Caregivers to the Elderly, 1987 and 1997 (Bethesda, Md.: National Alliance for Caregiving, June 1997).

18.   National Alliance for Caregiving, Caregiving in the U.S., National Alliance for Caregiving in collaboration with the AARP (November 2009), p. 5.

19.   "What Moves Americans to Move?" Census 2000, U.S. Census Bureau (http://usgovinfo.about.com/library/ weekly/aa060401a.htm).

20.   National Alliance for Caregiving, Caregiving in the U.S. (see note 18), p. 14.

21.   Linda K. Bledsoe, Sharon E. Moore, and Lott Collins, "Long Distance Caregiving:

An Evaluative Review of the Literature," Ageing International (New York: Springer Science, 2010); Beverly Koerin and Marcia Harrigan, "P.S. I Love You: Long Distance Caregiving," Journal of Gerontological Social Work 40, no. 1/2 (2003): 63–81.

22.   MetLife, Miles Away: The MetLife Study of Long-Distance Caregiving (Westport, Conn.: MetLife Mature Market Institute, July 2004).

23.   S. H. Matthews and T. T. Rosner, "Shared Filial Responsibility: The Family as the Primary Caregiver," Journal of Marriage and the Family 50, no. 1 (1998): 278–86; E. P. Stoller, L. E. Forster, and T. S. Duniho, "Systems of Parent Care within Sibling Networks," Research on Aging 14, no. 1 (1992): 472–92.

24.   E. Fuller-Thompson and M. Minkler, "Housing Issues and Realities Faced by Grandparent Caregivers Who Are Renters," Gerontologist 43, no. 1 (2003): 92–98.

25.   Continuing care retirement communities include "independent living" units for those who can still care for themselves; "assisted living" units for those who need some daily help with personal care; and "long-term- care" beds for those who are no longer able to take care of themselves.

26.   National Alliance for Caregiving, Caregiving in the U.S. (see note 18), p. 14.

27.   National Council on Aging, "Long-Term Services and Supports" (www.ncoa.org/independence-dignity/ long-term-services-supports.html).

28.   J. Keefe and others, "Caregivers' Aspirations, Realities, and Expectations: The CARE Tool," Journal of Applied Gerontology 27, no. 3 (2008): 286–308.

29.   Pew Research Center, "From the Age of Aquarius to the Age of Responsibility: Baby Boomers Approach Age 60, A Social Trends Report" (2005), pp. 10–13.

30.   Pew Research Center, Growing Old in America: Expectations vs. Reality, A Social and Demographic Trends Report (June 2009), p. 11.

31.   E. Papastavrou and others, "Caring for a Relative with Dementia: Family Caregiver Burden" (JAN Original Research, Blackwell Publishing, Ltd., 2007).

32.   Karen Donelan and others, "Challenged to Care: Informal Caregivers in a Changing Health Care System," Health Affairs 21, no. 4 (2002): 222–31 (http://content.healthaffairs.org/cgi/content/full/21/4/222).

33.   R. Johnson and J. Wiener, A Profile of Frail Older Americans and Their Caregivers, The Retirement Project, Occasional Paper 8 (Washington: Urban Institute, 2006). 136 THE FUTURE OF CHILDREN Ann Bookman and Delia Kimbrel

34.   Ibid, p. 24.

35.   MetLife, Broken Trust: Elders, Family, and Finances (Westport, Conn.: MetLife Mature Market Institute, 2009), p. 12.

36.   Joshua Hauser and Betty Kramer, "Family Caregivers in Palliative Care," Clinics in Geriatric Medicine 20, no. 4 (November 2004): 671–88.

37.   Luisa Margulies, My Mother's Hip: Lessons from the World of Elder Care (Philadelphia: Temple University Press, 2004).

38.   Kevin Brazil, Daryl Bainbridge, and Christine Rodriguez, "The Stress Process in Palliative Cancer Care: A Qualitative Study on Informal Caregiving and Its Implication for the Delivery of Care," American Journal of Hospice and Palliative Medicine 27, no. 2 (2010): 111–16.

39.   Arthur Kleinman, "On Caregiving: A Scholar Experiences the Moral Acts That Come Before—and Go Beyond—Modern Medicine," Harvard Magazine (July–August 2010):

27.

40. David O. Moberg, ed., Aging and Spirituality: Spiritual Dimensions of Aging Theory, Research, Practice, and Policy (Binghamton, N.Y.: Haworth Press, 2001).

41. M. Crowther and others, "Spiritual and Emotional Well-Being Tasks Associated with Elder Care," Geriatric Care Management Journal 13, no. 1 (Winter/Spring 2003): 15–21.

42. The Administration on Aging has a website to help families find an agency near where their elderly relative lives (www.eldercare.gov/Eldercare.NET/Public/Home.aspx).

43. T. Semla, "How to Improve Coordination of Care," Annals of Internal Medicine 148, no. 8 (April 15, 2008): 627–28.

44. Grif Alspach, "Handing Off Critically Ill Patients to Family Caregivers: What Are Your Best Practices?" Critical Care Nurse 29, no. 3 (2009): 12–22.

45. Bookman and Harrington, "Family Caregivers" (see note 14).

46. Laura Katz Olsen, The Not-So-Golden Years: Caregiving, the Frail Elderly, and the Long-Term Care Establishment (Lanham, Md.: Rowman & Littlefield Publishers, Inc., 2003), p. 98; Nancy R. Hooyman, "Research on Older Women: Where Is Feminism?" Gerontologist 39, no.1 (1999): 115–18.

47. National Alliance for Caregiving and AARP, Caregiving in the U.S.: A Focused Look at Those Caring for Someone Age 50 or Older (Washington, 2009), p. 22.

48. Kerstin Aumann and others, Working Family Caregivers of the Elderly: Everyday Realities and Wishes for Change (New York: Families and Work Institute, 2010), p. 2.

49. Ibid.

50. Lynn M. Martire and Mary Ann Parris Stephens, "Juggling Parent Care and Employment Responsibilities: The Dilemmas of Adult Daughter Caregivers in the Workforce," Sex Roles 48, no. 3/4 (2003): 167–73.

51. Olsen, The Not-So-Golden Years (see note 46).

52. Margaret B. Neal and Donna L. Wagner, "Working Caregivers: Issues, Challenges, and Opportunities for the Aging Network," National Family Caregiver Support Program Issue Brief (2002): 1–31. VOL. 21 / NO. 2 / FALL 2011 137 F

53. Susan C. Eaton, "Eldercare in the United States: Inadequate, Inequitable, but Not a Lost Cause," Feminist Economics 11, no. 2 (2005): 37–51; MetLife Mature Market Institute, Employer Costs for Working Caregivers (Washington: MetLife Mature Market Institute and National Alliance for Caregivers, 1997).

54. Karen Bullock, Sybil L. Crawford, and Sharon L. Tennstedt, "Employment and Caregiving: Exploration of African American Caregivers," Social Work 48, no. 2 (2003): 150–62.

55. MetLife, MetLife Study of Working Caregivers and Employer Health Costs (Westport, Conn.: National Alliance for Caregiving and MetLife Mature Market Institute, February 2010).

56. Peter P. Vitaliano, Jianping Zhang, and James M. Scanlan, "Is Caregiving Hazardous to One's Physical Health? A Meta-Analysis," Psychological Bulletin 129, no. 6 (2003): 946–72.

57. Martin Pinquart and Silvia Sörensen, "Gender Differences, Caregiver Stressors, Social Resources, and Health: An Updated Meta-Analysis," Journals of Gerontology Series B: Psychological Sciences & Social Sciences 61, no. 1 (2006): 33–45.

58. Ibid.

59.   Sara Torres, "Barriers to Mental-Health Care Access Faced by Hispanic Elderly," in Servicing Minority Elders in the Twenty-First Century, edited by Mary L. Wykle and Amasa B.
Ford (New York: Springer, 1999), pp. 200–18.

60.   Sarah J. Yarry, Elizabeth K. Stevens, and T. J. McCallum, "Cultural Influences on Spousal Caregiving," American Society on Aging 31, no. 3 (2007): 24–30.

61.   James Jackson, "African American Aged," in the Encyclopedia of Aging, 2nd ed., edited by George L. Maddox (New York: Springer, 1995), pp. 30–80; Sharon L. Tennstedt, BeiHung Chang, and Melvin Delgado, "Patterns of Long-Term Care: A Comparison of Puerto Rican, African-American, and Non-Latino White Elders," Journal of Gerontological Social Work 30, no. 1/2 (1998): 179–99.

62.   Sue Levkoff, Becca Levy, and Patricia Flynn Weitzmann, "The Role of Religion and Ethnicity in the Help Seeking of Family Caregivers of Elders with Alzheimer's Disease and Related Disorders," Journal of Cross- Cultural Gerontology 14, no. 4 (1999): 335.

63.   Martin Pinquart and Silvia Sörensen, "Associations of Stressors and Uplifts of Caregiving with Caregiver Burden and Depressive Mood: A Meta-Analysis," Journals of Gerontology Series B: Psychological Sciences & Social Sciences 58B, no. 2 (2003): 112; D. W. Coon and others, "Well-Being, Appraisal, and Coping in Latina and Caucasian Female Dementia Caregivers: Findings from the REACH Study," Aging & Mental Health 8, no. 4 (2004): 330–45.

64.   W. E. Haley and others, "Well-Being, Appraisal, and Coping in African-American and Caucasian Dementia Caregivers: Findings from the REACH Study," Aging &Mental Health 8, no. 4 (2004): 316–29; Coon and others, "Well-Being, Appraisal, and Coping in Latina and Caucasian Female Dementia Caregivers" (see note 63).

65.   Tennstedt, Chang, and Delgado, "Patterns of Long-Term Care" (see note 61).

66.   Catherine Hagan Hennessey and Robert John, "American Indian Family Caregivers'
Perceptions of Burden and Needed Support Services," Journal of Applied Gerontology 15, no. 3 (1996): 275–93. 138 THE FUTURE OF CHILDREN Ann Bookman and Delia Kimbrel

67.   Martin Pinquart and Silvia Sörensen, "Ethnic Differences in Stressors, Resources, and Psychological Outcomes of Family Caregiving: A Meta-Analysis," Gerontologist 45, no. 1 (2005): 90–106; M. R. Janevic and M. C. Connell, "Racial, Ethnic, and Cultural Differences in the Dementia Caregiving Experience: Recent Finding," Gerontologist 41, no. 3 (2001): 334–47.

68.   Karen I. Fredriksen-Goldsen and Nancy Farwell, "Dual Responsibilities among Black, Hispanic, Asian, and White Employed Caregivers," Journal of Gerontological Social Work 43, no. 4 (2004): 25–44.

69.   Peggye Dilworth-Anderson, Ishan Canty Williams, and Brent E. Gibson, "Issues of Race, Ethnicity, and Culture in Caregiving Research: A 20-Year Review (1980–2000)," Gerontologist 42, no. 2 (2002): 237–72.

70.   Tatjana Meschede, Thomas M. Shapiro, and Jennifer Wheary, Living Longer on Less: The New Economic Insecurity of Seniors (Institute on Assets and Social Policy and Demos, 2009).

71.   Administration on Aging, A Profile of Older Americans: 2009 (www.aoa.gov/AoAroot/Aging_Statistics/ Profile/2009/docs/2009profile_508.pdf).

72.   Deborah M. Merrill, Caring for Elderly Parents: Juggling Work, Family, and Caregiving in Middle and Working Class Families (Westport: Auburn House, 1997), pp. 13–15.

73. Ibid.

74. Rachel F. Boaz, "Full-Time Employment and Informal Caregiving in the 1980s," Medical Care 34, no. 6 (1996): 524–36.

75. Robyn Stone, Gail Lee Cafferata, and Judith Sangl, "Caregivers of the Frail Elderly: A National Profile," Gerontologist 27, no. 5 (1987): 616–26.

76. Wagner, Comparative Analysis of Caregiver Data for Caregivers to the Elderly, 1987 and 1997 (see note 17), p. 2.

77. MetLife, MetLife Study of Working Caregivers and Employer Health Costs (see note 55).

78. Margaret B. Neal and others, Balancing Work and Caregiving for Children, Adults, and Elders (Newbury Park, Calif.: Sage, 1993); Urie Bronfenbrenner and others, The State of Americans: This Generation and the Next (New York: Free Press, 1996); J. L. Gibeau, J. W. Anastas, and P. J. Larson, "Breadwinners, Caregivers, and Employers: New Alliances in an Aging America," Employee Benefits Journal 12, no. 3 (1987): 6–10; Andrew E. Scharlach, "Caregiving and Employment: Competing or Complementary Roles?" Gerontologist 34, no. 3 (1994): 378–85.

79. Evercare, Family Caregivers—What They Spend, What They Sacrifice (Minnetonka, Minn.: 2007), p. 21.

80. R. Schutltz and S. Beach, "Caregiving as a Risk Factor for Mortality: The Caregiver Health Effects Study," Journal of the American Medical Association 282, no. 23 (1999): 2215– 19; R. Schutlz,, P. Visintainer, and G. M. Williamson, "Psychiatric and Physical Morbidity Effect of Caregiving," Journal of Gerontology 45, no. 5 (1990): 181–91.

81. National Alliance for Caregiving and the National Center for Women and Aging at Brandeis University, The MetLife Juggling Act Study: Balancing Caregiving with Work and the Costs Involved (New York: The MetLife Mature Market Institute, 1999). VOL. 21 / NO. 2 / FALL 2011 139 Families and Elder Care in the Twenty-First Century

82. Society for Human Resource Management (SHRM), 2007 Employee Benefits Survey (Alexandria, Va.: 2007).

83. Hewitt Associates, Work/Life Benefits Provided by Major U.S. Employers in 2003– 2004 (Lincolnshire, Ill.: 2003)

84. SHRM, 2007 Employee Benefits Survey (see note 82).

85. Ellen Galinsky and James T. Bond, The Impact of the Recession on Employers (New York: Families and Work Institute, 2009), p. 7 (www.familiesandwork.org/site/research/reports/Recession2009.pdf).

86. Allarde Dembe and others, "Employer Perceptions of Elder Care Assistance Programs," Journal of Workplace Behavioral Health 23, no. 4 (2008): 360.

87. SHRM, 2007 Employee Benefits Survey (see note 82).

88. Donna Wagner and Gail Hunt, "The Use of Workplace Eldercare Programs by Employed Caregivers," Research on Aging 16, no. 1 (March 1994): 69–84.

89. Dembe and others, "Employer Perceptions of Elder Care Assistance Programs" (see note 86), p. 371.

90. Ibid., p. 373.

91. Terry Bond and others, The National Study of Employers: Highlights of Findings (New York: Families and Work Institute, 2006).

92. J. L. Glass and A. Finley, "Coverage and Effectiveness of Family Responsive Workplace Policies," Human Resources Management Review 12, no. 3 (Autumn 2002): 313–37.

93. Marcie Pitt-Catsouphes, Christina Matz-Costa, and Elyssa Besen, Age and Generations: Understanding Experiences at the Workplace (Chestnut Hill, Mass.: Boston College, 2009), p. 17.

94. Ibid.

95. Bond, The National Study of Employers (see note 91).

96. Muriel Gillick, The Denial of Aging: Perpetual Youth, Eternal Life, and Other Dangerous Fantasies (Harvard University Press, 2006), pp. 4, 6.

97. Ellen Galinsky, Dana Friedman, and C. Hernandez, The Corporate Reference Guide to Work-Family Programs (New York: Families and Work Institute, 1991).

98. Tamara Haraven, "The Changing Patterns of Family Life as They Affect the Aged," Families and Older Persons: Policy Research and Practice, edited by G. K. Maddox, I. C. Siegler, and D. G. Blazer (Durham, N.C.: Duke University Center for the Study of Aging and Human Development, 1980), pp. 31–41.

99. Nancy Folbre, The Invisible Heart (New York: The New Press, 2001), p. 102.

100. Centers for Medicare and Medicaid Services, "National Health Accounts" (http://cms.hhs.gov/statistics/nhe).

101. Brenda Spillman and Peter Kemper, "Lifetime Patterns of Payment for Nursing Home Care," Medical Care 33, no. 3 (1995): 280–96.

102. Centers for Medicare and Medicaid Services, Brief Summaries of Medicare and Medicaid, 2010 (www.cms.gov/MedicareProgramRatesStats/downloads/MedicareMedicaidSummaries2010.pdf). 140 THE FUTURE OF CHILDREN Ann Bookman and Delia Kimbrel

103. Carol Levine, ed., Always on Call: When Illness Turns Families into Caregivers (New York: United Hospital Fund, 2004), p. 137.

104. L. W. Kaye, "The Adequacy of the Older Americans Act Home Care Mandate: A Front Line View from Three Programs," Home Health Care Service Quarterly 5, no. 1 (Spring 1984): 75–87.

105. T. Burns and others, "Home Treatment for Mental Health Problems: A Systemic Review," Health Technology Assessment 5, no. 15 (2001): 1–139.

106. Jo Harris-Wehling and others, Real Problems, Real People: An Evaluation of the Long-Term Care Ombudsman Programs of the Older Americans Act (Washington: Division of Health Care Services, Institute of Medicine, 1995).

107. Commission on Leave, A Workable Balance: A Report to Congress on Family and Medical Leave Policies (Washington: U.S. Department of Labor, May 1996).

108. David Cantor and others, Balancing the Needs of Families and Employers: Family and Medical Leave Surveys (Bethesda, Md.: Westat, 2001).

109. Jane Waldfogel, "Family and Medical Leave: Evidence from the 2000 Surveys," Monthly Labor Review 124, no. 9 (September 2001): 17–23.

110. Ruth Milkman and Eileen Applebaum, "Leaves That Pay: Employer and Worker Experiences with Paid Family Leave in California" (Center for Research on Economic Policy, January 2011), pp. 1–36.

111.   Theda Skocpol, Protecting Soldiers and Mothers: The Political Origins of Social Policy in the United States (Harvard University Press, 1992), pp. 46–47.

112.   Stephanie Whittier, Andrew Scharlach, and Teresa S. Dal Santo, "Availability of Caregiver Support Services: Implications for Implementation of the National Family Caregiver Support Program," Journal of Aging and Social Policy 17, no. 1 (2005): 45–62.

113.   In 2006, Congress passed the "Lifespan Respite Care Act" (Public Law 109-442), but no funds have been allocated for implementation.

C.

Why a Family Support System is Important for the Elderly

SEPTEMBER 15, 2021

|IN **LIBERTY HOME CARE AND HOSPICE**
|BY **LIBERTY HOMECARE AND HOSPICE**

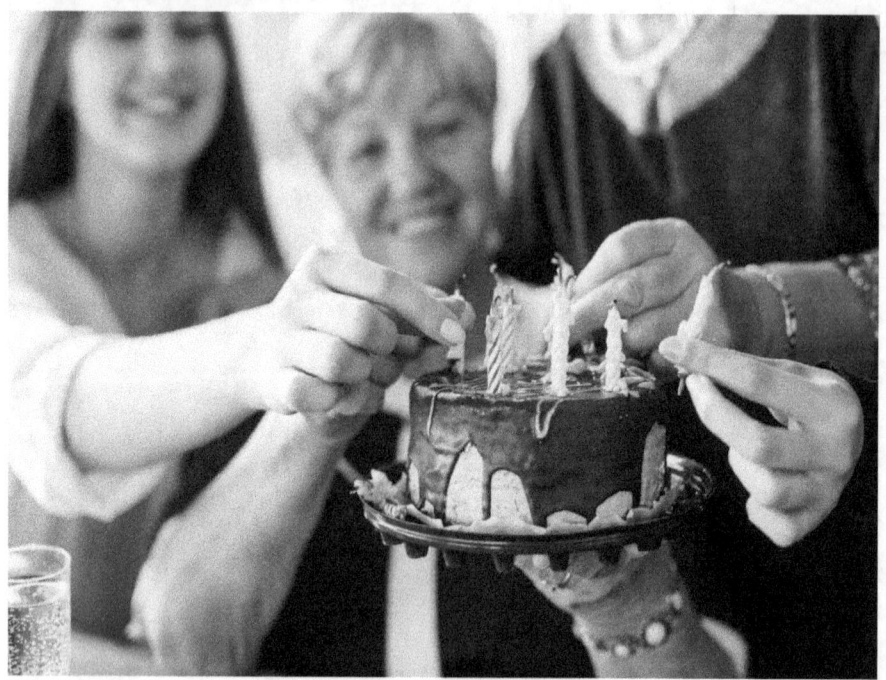

As people age, having a family support system is crucial for the elderly. A support system provides a social network, helps improve their loved one's health, and can even extend their life compared to older adults without any friends or family. Let's take a look at why a family support system is beneficial for the elderly.

A Direct Connection Between Family and Health

A United States Aging Survey found that 30 percent of seniors believe staying connected to family and friends is a main concern. The survey found that most seniors believe that maintaining relationships with family and friends is more important than having financial support. Aside from older adults' views, studies have shown a direct connection between an older adult's health and their relationship with family. Indeed, family is important for the elderly's mental, physical, and social health.

What Are the Benefits of a Family Support System for the Elderly?

1. Longer Life Expectancy

When older adults maintain social connections with their family members, this can increase their life expectancy compared to those that are socially isolated. It may not be an obvious benefit, but a family's presence can improve their overall health in their remaining years. This is also true for those with dementia.

2. Stronger Immune System

Older adults that have a family support system and regularly connect with others typically have stronger immune systems. This is a major benefit, especially since older adults tend to have weaker immune systems as they age. In turn, a healthier immune system will be better equipped to fight off illnesses that older adults come in contact with.

3. Better Mental Health

Another benefit for seniors that stay close with family is having improved <u>mental</u> <u>health</u> compared to those that aren't close to loved ones. It's important for older adults to socialize with their family and to be reminded that they are loved and valued. This can help seniors be less likely to suffer from mental illnesses like depression.

4. Better Brain Health

Older adults who stay socially connected also benefit from having higher levels of cognitive function. Studies have shown that those that enjoyed participating in social activities were more likely to have better memory and thinking skills. On the other hand, older adults that did not enjoy socializing experienced a decrease in their cognitive health.

5. A Family Support System

Like any family, the type of support and interactions change overtime. A parent that once supported and took care of their child will eventually have the roles reversed as the adult child cares for and supports the aging parent. This is a normal part of life.

For many aging parents, financial support is necessary to receive the medical care required as they age. When their family is able to offer this support, this can melt away some of the <u>stress</u> that an older adult may feel. This is important, especially when stress can weaken an older adult's already weakened immune system.

Additionally, emotional support is another major benefit of having a support system. It helps to have someone to talk to and listen to them about their good and bad days. This shows them that their family cares, which can have a positive impact on their outlook on life.

Another type of support is to help older adults perform daily activities, such as cleaning their house, going shopping, or even cooking. If an older adult has a bigger family, the family can take turns helping the older adult out. These simple acts can make a big difference in helping seniors not feel alone.

6. Friendships Are Important Too

Since not every older adult has family near them, they can still benefit from social connections and support from old and new friends. Studies have shown that having strong social connections has a positive benefit to seniors' health, whether that is with friends or family.

If an older adult wants to make new friends, there are quite a few tips to achieve this great goal. Older adults can visit their local pool, volunteer at a local organization, take a community class for seniors, or join a gym. There are plenty of options to discover new friendships and stay connected with others.

We hope this article was helpful, especially if you have an older adult in your life. A family support system isn't just beneficial, it's crucial for the elderly's mental, physical, and emotional health and well-being. For those that do not have nearby family, a close group of friends can still provide the same benefits. Contact **Liberty HomeCare and Hospice Services** today to learn more about our **home care**, hospice care, and palliative care designed to help your loved one's achieve their highest quality of life in the place they love – their homes.

6.5 Problems Facing Older Americans

Learning Objectives

1. Present a brief sociodemographic profile of the US elderly.
2. Discuss the several problems experienced by the US elderly.
3. Describe how the social attitudes of older Americans generally differ from those of younger Americans.

We now turn our attention to older people in the United States. We first sketch a demographic profile of our elderly and then examine some of the problems they face because of their age and because of ageism.

Who Are the Elderly?

Table 6.2 "Demographic Composition of the Elderly, 2010" presents the demographic composition of Americans aged 65 or older. Slightly more than half the elderly are 65–74 years of age, and about 57 percent are female, reflecting males' shorter life spans as discussed earlier. About 80 percent of the elderly are non-Latino whites, compared to about 66 percent in the population as a whole; 8.6 percent are African American, compared to about 13 percent of the population; and 7.0 percent are Latino, compared to 15 percent of the population. The greater proportion of whites among the elderly and lower proportions of African Americans and Latinos reflects these groups' life expectancy differences discussed earlier and also their differences in birth rates.

Table 6.2 Demographic Composition of the Elderly, 2010

Age	
65–74 years	52.3%
75–84 years	33.4%
85 years and over	14.3%
Gender	
Female	56.9%
Male	43.1%
Race and/or ethnicity*	

White, non-Latino	80.1%
African American	8.6%
Latino	7.0%
Asian/Pacific Islander	3.5%
Amer. Ind., Esk., Aleut.	0.6%
Two or more races	0.7%
Living in poverty	9.0%
Marital status	
Married	57.6%
Widowed	28.1%

Divorced	10.0%
Never married	4.3%

Years of school completed

0–8 years	10.2%
1–3 years of high school	10.3%
High school graduate	36.4%
1–3 years of college	20.6%
College graduate	22.5%

Labor force participation

Employed	16.2%

Unemployed	1.2%
Not in labor force	82.6%

Household income*

Under $15,000	18.8%
$15,000–$24,999	20.7%
$25,000–$34,999	15.4%
$35,000–49,999	15.1%
$50,000–$74,999	14.2%
$75,000–$99,999	6.5%
$100,000 and over	9.4%

Source: Data from US Census Bureau. (2012). *Statistical abstract of the United States: 2012.* Washington, DC: US Government Printing Office. Retrieved from http://www.census.gov/compendia/statab.

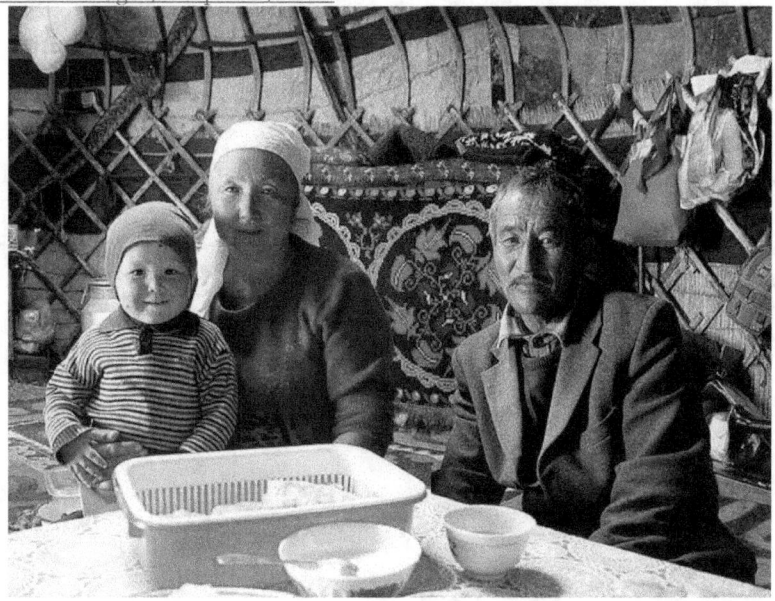

The lower proportions of African Americans and Latinos among the elderly partly reflect these groups' lower life expectancies.
Evgeni Zotov – Grandparents – CC BY-NC-ND 2.0.

The percentage of elders living in poverty is 9.0, compared to 15.1 percent of the entire population. **Although most elders have fixed incomes, the fact that their family size is usually one or two means that they are less likely than younger people to live in poverty. In fact, today's elderly are financially much better off than their grandparents were, thanks to Social Security, Medicare (the federal health insurance program for older Americans), pensions, and their own assets.** We will revisit the health and financial security of elders a little later.

Turning to education, about 22 percent of the elderly are college graduates, compared to about 29 percent of the population as a whole. This difference reflects the fact that few people went to college when today's elderly were in their late teens and early twenties. However, it is still true that today's elders are better educated than any previous generation of elders. Future generations of the elderly will be even better educated than those now.

74

While most elders are retired and no longer in the labor force, about 16 percent do continue to work (see Table 6.2 "Demographic Composition of the Elderly, 2010"). These seniors tend to be in good health and to find their jobs psychologically satisfying. Compared to younger workers, they miss fewer days of work for health or other reasons and are less likely to quit their jobs for other opportunities (Sears, 2009).

Although we emphasized earlier that many older Americans do not fit the negative image with which they are portrayed, it is still true that they face special problems because of their age and life circumstances and because of ageism. We discuss some of these here.

Physical and Mental Health

Perhaps the problem that comes most readily to mind is health, or, to be more precise, poor health. It is true that many older people remain in good health and are fully able to function mentally and physically (Rowe et al., 2010). Still, the biological and psychological effects of aging do lead to greater physical and mental health problems among the elderly than in younger age groups, as we briefly discussed earlier. These problems are reflected in responses to the General Social Survey (GSS) question, "Would you say your own health, in general, is excellent, good, fair, or poor?" Figure 6.6 "Age and Self-Reported Health" shows that the elderly are more likely than the nonelderly to report that their health is only fair or poor.

Figure 6.6 Age and Self-Reported Health

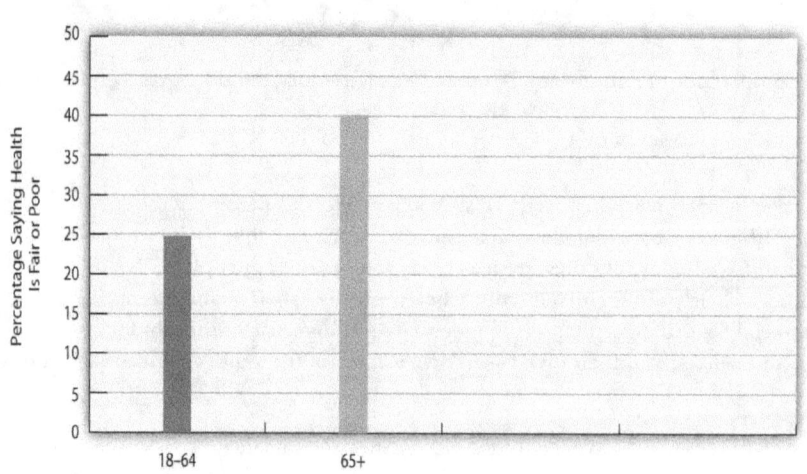

Source: Data from General Social Survey. (2010). Retrieved from
http://sda.berkeley.edu/cgibin/hsda?harcsda+gss10.

The elderly's perception of their own health is supported by government estimates of chronic health conditions for older Americans. Of all people aged 65 or older not living in a nursing home or other institution, almost 50 percent have arthritis, 56 percent have high blood pressure,

32 percent have heart disease, 35 percent have hearing loss, 18 percent have vision problems, and 19 percent have diabetes (these numbers add up to more than 100 percent as people may have several health conditions) (Federal Interagency Forum on Aging-Related Statistics, 2010). These rates are much higher than those for younger age groups.

The elderly also suffer from dementia, including Alzheimer's disease, which affects almost 13 percent of people 65 or older (Alzheimer's Association, 2009). Another mental health problem is depression, which affects almost 15 percent of people 65 or older. Because of mental or physical disability, about two-thirds of all people 65 or older need help with at least one "daily living" activity, such as preparing a meal (Federal Interagency Forum on Aging-Related Statistics, 2010).

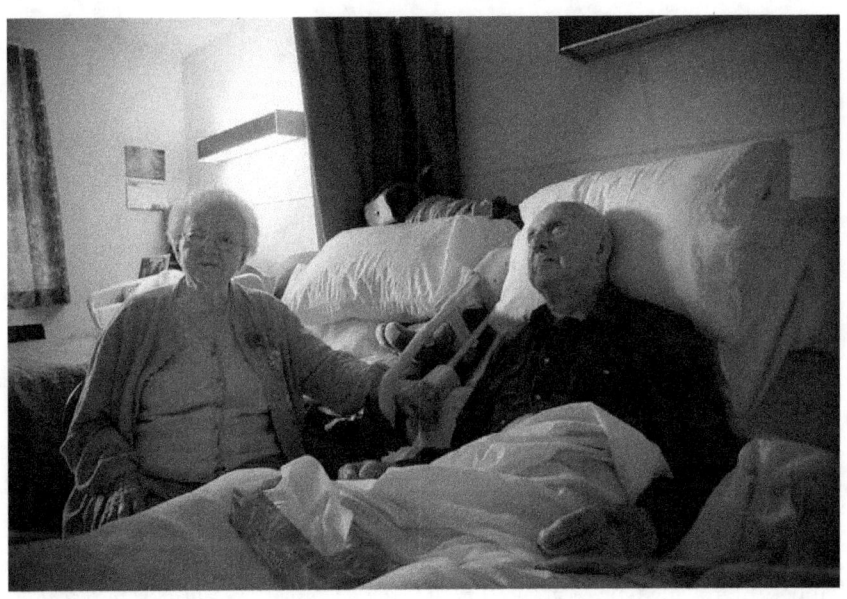

Older people visit the doctor and hospital more often than younger people. Partly for this reason, adequate health care for the elderly is of major importance. Ted Van Pelt – The Coopers – CC BY 2.0.

If the elderly have more health problems, then adequate care for them is of major importance. They visit the doctor and hospital more often than their middle-aged counterparts. Medicare covers about one-half of their health-care costs; this is a substantial amount of coverage but still forces many seniors to pay thousands of dollars annually themselves. Some physicians and other health-care providers do not accept Medicare "assignment," meaning that the patient must pay an even higher amount. Moreover, Medicare pays little or nothing for long-term care in nursing homes and other institutions and for mental health services. All these factors mean that older Americans can still face high medical expenses or at least pay high premiums for private health insurance.

In addition, Medicare costs have risen rapidly along with other health-care costs. Medicare expenditures soared from about $37 billion in 1980 to more than $500 billion today (see Figure

6.7 "Medicare Expenditures, 1980–2010"). As the population continues to age and as health-care costs continue to rise, Medicare expenses will continue to rise as well, making it increasingly difficult to find the money to finance Medicare.

Figure 6.7 Medicare Expenditures, 1980–2010

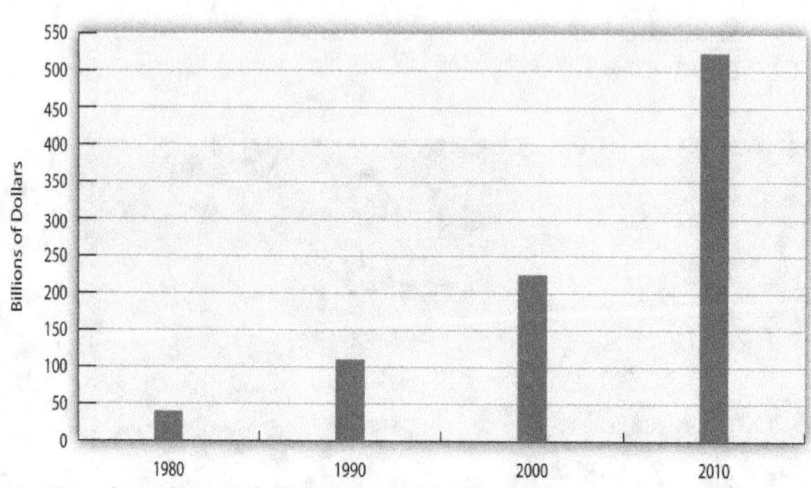

Source: Data from Centers for Medicare and Medicaid Services. (n.d.). National health expenditure data. Retrieved from http://www.hhs.gov.

Nursing Home Care

While most older Americans live by themselves or with their families, a small minority live in group settings. A growing type of group setting is the *continuous care retirement community*, a setting of private rooms, apartments, and/or condominiums that offers medical and practical care to those who need it. In some such communities, residents eat their meals together, while in others they cook for themselves. Usually these communities offer above-average recreational facilities and can be very expensive, as some require a lifetime contract or at least monthly fees that can run into the thousands of dollars.

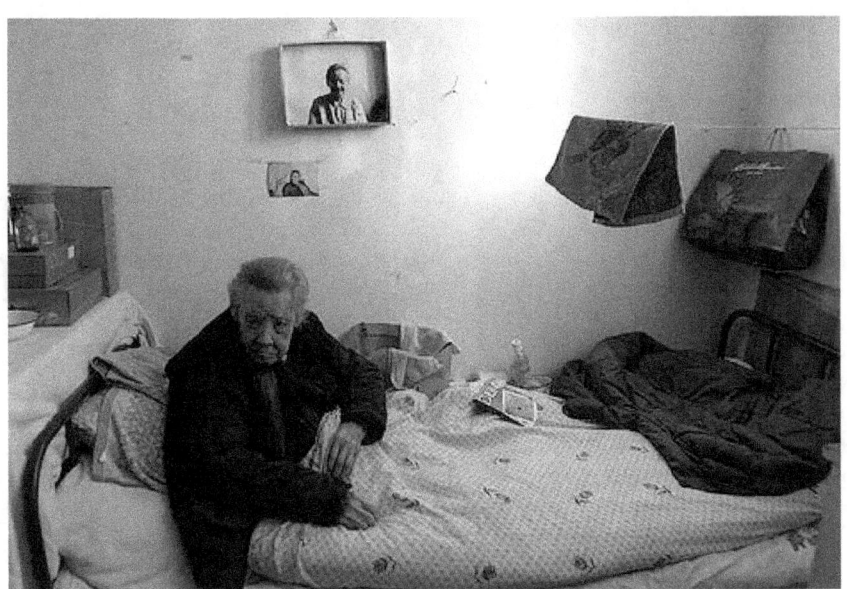

Nursing homes are often understaffed to save costs and are also generally not subject to outside inspection. These conditions help contribute to the neglect of nursing home residents. Sheila – <u>Christian Nursing Home</u> – CC BY-NC-ND 2.0.

For elders who need high-level medical care or practical support, nursing homes are the primary option. About 16,100 nursing homes exist, and 3.9 percent of Americans 65 or older live in them (Federal Interagency Forum on Aging-Related Statistics, 2010). About three-fourths of all nursing home residents are women. Almost all residents receive assistance in bathing and showering, 80 percent receive help in using the bathroom, and one-third receive help in eating.

As noted earlier, Medicare does not pay for long-term institutional care for most older Americans. Because nursing home care costs at least $70,000 yearly, residents can quickly use up all their assets and then, ironically, become eligible for payments from *Medicaid*, the federal insurance program for people with low incomes.

If one problem of nursing homes is their expense, another problem is the quality of care they provide. Because their residents are typically in poor physical and/or mental health, their care must be the best possible, as they can do little to help themselves if their care is substandard. As more people enter nursing homes in the years ahead, the quality of nursing home care will become even more important. Yet there is much evidence that nursing home care is often substandard and is replete with neglect and abuse (DeHart, Webb, & Cornman, 2009).

Financial Security and Employment

Earlier we noted that the elderly are less likely than younger age groups to live in poverty and that their financial status is much better than that of previous generations of older people. One reason for this is Social Security: If Social Security did not exist, the poverty rate of the elderly would be 45 percent, or five times higher than the actual rate (Kerby, 2012). Without Social Security, then, nearly half of all people 65 or older would be living in official poverty, and this rate would be even much higher for older women and older persons of color. However, this brief summary of their economic well-being obscures some underlying problems (Carr, 2010; Crawthorne, 2008).

First, recall Chapter 2 "Poverty"'s discussion of *episodic poverty*, which refers to the drifting of many people into and out of poverty as their jobs and other circumstances change. Once they become poor, older people are more likely than younger ones to *stay* poor, as younger people have more job and other opportunities to move out of poverty. Recall also that the official poverty rate obscures the fact that many people live just above it and are "near poor." This is especially true of the elderly, who, if hit by large medical bills or other expenses, can hardly afford to pay them.

Second, the extent of older Americans' poverty varies by sociodemographic factors and is much worse for some groups than for others (Carr, 2010). Older women, for example, are more likely than older men to live in poverty for at least two reasons. Because women earn less than men and are more likely to take time off from work during their careers, they have lower monthly Social Security benefits than men and smaller pensions from their employers. As well, women outlive men and thus use up their savings. Racial and ethnic disparities also exist among the elderly, reflecting poverty disparities in the entire population, as older people of color are much more likely than older whites to live in poverty (Carr, 2010). Among women 65 and older, 9 percent of whites live in poverty, compared to 27 percent of African Americans, 12 percent of Asians, and 21 percent of Hispanics.

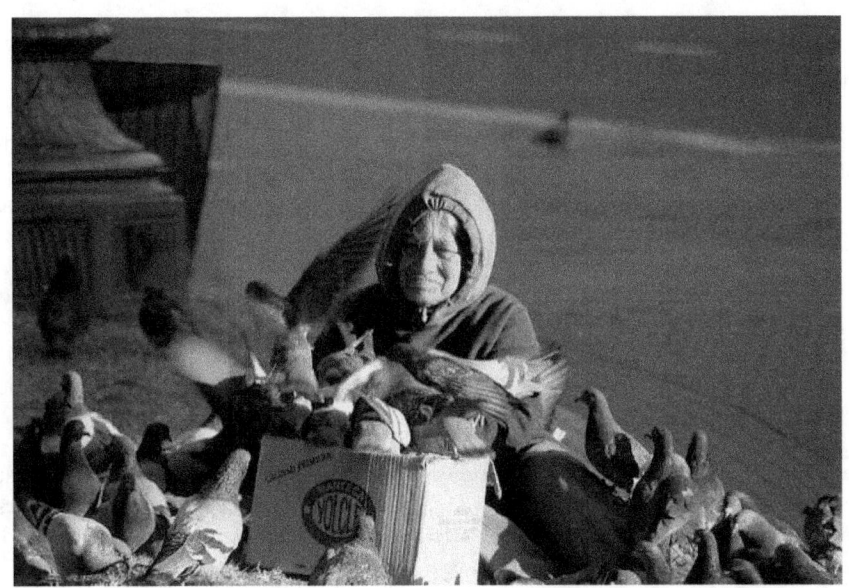

Older women are more likely than older men to live in poverty.
Christian Haugen – <u>Old woman feeding the pigeon</u> – CC BY 2.0.

Third, monthly Social Security benefits are tied to people's earnings before retirement; the higher the earnings, the higher the monthly benefit. Thus a paradox occurs: People who earn low wages will get lower Social Security benefits after they retire, even though they need *higher* benefits to make up for their lower earnings. In this manner, the income inequality that exists before retirement continues to exist after it.

This paradox reflects a wider problem involving Social Security. However helpful it might be in aiding older Americans, the aid it provides lags far behind comparable programs in other wealthy Western nations (see <u>Note 6.27 "Lessons from Other Societies"</u>). Social Security payments are low enough that almost one-third of the elderly who receive no other income assistance live in official poverty. For all these reasons, Social Security is certainly beneficial for many older Americans, but it remains inadequate compared to what other nations provide.

Lessons from Other Societies

4. Aging Policy and Programs in the Netherlands and Sweden

A few years ago, AARP assessed quality-of-life issues for older people and the larger society in sixteen wealthy democracies (the nations of North America and Western Europe, along with Australia and Japan). Each nation was rated (on a scale of 1–5, with 5 being the highest score) on seventeen criteria, including life expectancy, health care for the elderly, pension coverage, and age-discrimination laws. Of the sixteen nations, the Netherlands ranked first, with a total score of 64, while Italy ranked last, with a score of 48; the United States was thirteenth, with a score of 50. Despite its immense wealth, then, the United States lagged behind most other democracies.

Because a "perfect" score would have been 85 (17 × 5), even the Netherlands fell short of an ideal quality of life as measured by the AARP indicators.

Why did the United States not rank higher? The experience of the Netherlands and Sweden, both of which have longer life expectancies than the United States, points to some possible answers. In the Netherlands, everyone at age 65 receives a full pension that does not depend on how much money they earned while they were working, and everyone thus gets the same amount. This amount is larger than the average American gets, because Social Security does depend on earnings and many people earned fairly low amounts during their working years. As a result, Dutch elderly are much less likely than their American counterparts to be poor. The Dutch elderly (and also the nonelderly) have generous government insurance for medical problems and for nursing home care; this financial help is much higher than older Americans obtain through Medicare.

As one example, the AARP article mentioned an elderly Dutch woman who had cancer surgery and thirty-two chemotherapy treatments, for which she paid nothing. In the United States, the chemotherapy treatments would have cost at least $30,000. Medicare would have covered only 80 percent of this amount, leaving a patient to pay $6,000.

The Netherlands also helps its elderly in other ways. One example is that about one-fourth of that nation's elderly receive regular government-subsidized home visits by health-care professionals and/or housekeepers; this practice enables the elderly to remain independent and avoid having to enter a nursing home. In another example, the elderly also receive seven days of free riding on the nation's rail system.

Sweden has a home-care visitation program that is similar to the Netherlands' program. Many elderly are visited twice a day by a care assistant who helps them bathe and dress in the morning and go to bed at night. The care assistant also regularly cleans their residence and takes them out for exercise. The Swedish government pays about 80 percent of the costs of this assistance and subsidizes the remaining cost for elderly who cannot afford it. Like the Netherlands' program, Sweden's program helps the elderly to remain independent and live at home rather than enter a nursing institution.

Compared to the United States, then, other democracies generally provide their elderly less expensive or free health care, greater financial support during their retirement, and home visits by health-care professionals and other assistants. In these and other ways, these other governments encourage "active aging." Adoption of similar policies in the United States would improve the lives of older Americans and perhaps prolong their life spans.

Sources: Edwards, 2004; Hartlapp & Schmid, 2008; Ney, 2005

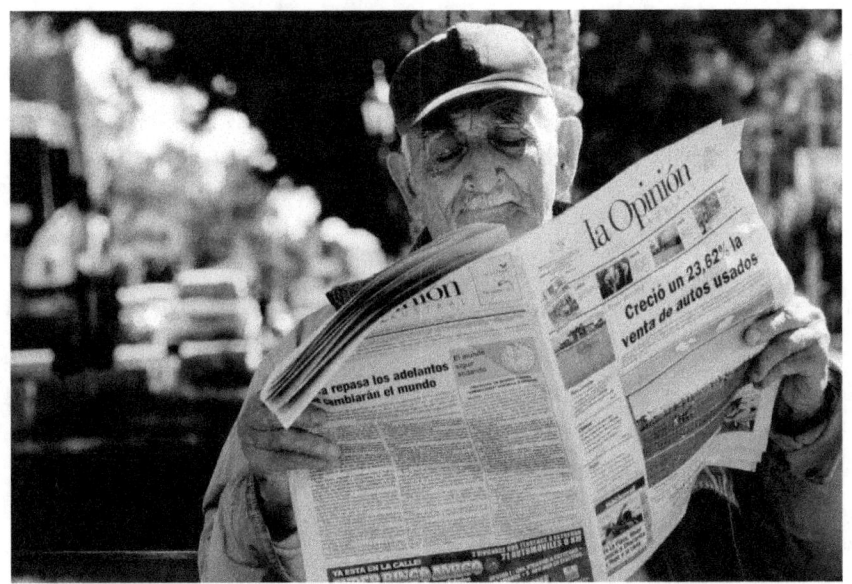

Older people who want to work may have trouble finding employment because of age discrimination and other factors.

Workplace Ageism

Older Americans also face problems in employment. Recall that about 16 percent of seniors remain employed. Other elders may wish to work but are retired or unemployed because several obstacles make it difficult for them to find jobs. First, many workplaces do not permit the parttime working arrangements that many seniors favor. Second, and as the opening news story indicated, the rise in high-tech jobs means that older workers would need to be retrained for many of today's jobs, and few retraining programs exist. Third, although federal law prohibits age discrimination in employment, it exists anyway, as employers do not think older people are "up to" the job, even though the evidence indicates they are good, productive workers (Berger, 2009; Roscigno, 2010). Finally, earnings above a certain level reduce Social Security benefits before full retirement age, leading some older people to avoid working at all or to at least limit their hours. All these obstacles lead seniors to drop out of the labor force or to remain unemployed (Gallo, Brand, Teng, Leo-Summers, & Byers, 2009).

Age discrimination in the workplace merits some further discussion. According to sociologist Vincent J. Roscigno (2010), survey evidence suggests that more than half of older workers have experienced or observed age discrimination in the workplace, and more than 80 percent of older workers have experienced or observed jokes, disrespect, or other prejudicial comments about old age. Roscigno notes that workplace ageism receives little news media attention and has also been neglected by social scientists. This is so despite the related facts that ageism in the workplace is common and that the older people who experience this discrimination suffer financial loss and emotional problems. Roscigno (2010, p. 17) interviewed several victims of age discrimination and later wrote, "Many conveyed fear of defaulting on mortgages or being unable to pay for their children's college after being pushed out of their jobs. Others expressed anger and insecurity over the loss of affordable health insurance or pension benefits…Just as prevalent and somewhat surprising to me in these discussions were the less-tangible, yet deeper socialpsychological and emotional costs that social science research has established for racial discrimination or sexual harassment, for instance, but are only now being considered in relation to older workers."

One of the people Roscigno interviewed was a maintenance worker who was laid off after more than two decades of working for his employer. This worker was both hurt and angry. "They now don't want to pay me my pension," he said. "I was a good worker for them and always did everything they asked. I went out of my way to help train people and make everything run smoothly, so everybody was happy and it was a good place to work. And now this is what I get, like I never really mattered to them. It's just not right" (Roscigno, 2010, p. 17).

Bereavement and Social Isolation

"We all need someone we can lean on," as a famous Rolling Stones song goes. Most older Americans do have adequate social support networks, which, as we saw earlier, are important for their well-being. However, a significant minority of elders live alone and do not see friends and relatives as often as they wish. Bereavement takes a toll, as elders who might have been married for many years suddenly find themselves living alone. Here a gender difference again exists. Because women outlive men and are generally younger than their husbands, they are three times more likely than men (42 percent compared to 13 percent) to be widowed and thus much more likely to live alone (see Table 6.3 "Living Arrangements of Noninstitutionalized Older Americans, 2010").

Table 6.3 Living Arrangements of Noninstitutionalized Older Americans, 2010

	Men (%)	Women (%)
Living alone	19	41
Living with spouse	70	37
Other arrangement	11	21

Source: Data from Administration on Aging. (2011). A profile of older Americans: 2011. Retrieved from http://www.aoa.gov/aoaroot/aging_statistics/Profile/2011/docs/2011profile.pdf.

Many elders have at least one adult child living within driving distance, and such children are an invaluable resource. At the same time, however, some elders have no children, because either they have outlived their children or they never had any. As baby boomers begin reaching their older years, more of them will have no children because they were more likely than previous generations to not marry and/or to not have children if they did marry. Baby boomers thus face a relative lack of children to help them when they enter their "old-old" years (Leland, 2010).

Bereavement is always a difficult experience, but because so many elders lose a spouse, it is a particular problem in their lives. The grief that usually follows bereavement can last several years and, if it becomes extreme, can involve anxiety, depression, guilt, loneliness, and other problems. Of all these problems, loneliness is perhaps the most common and the most difficult to overcome.

Elder Abuse

Some seniors fall prey to their own relatives who commit elder abuse against them. Such abuse involves one or more of the following: physical or sexual violence, psychological or emotional abuse, neglect of care, or financial exploitation (Novak, 2012). Accurate data are hard to come by since few elders report their abuse, but estimates say that at least 10 percent of older Americans have suffered at least one form of abuse, amounting to hundreds of thousands of cases annually. However, few of these cases come to the attention of the police or other authorities (National Center on Elder Abuse, 2010).

Although we may never know the actual extent of elder abuse, it poses a serious health problem for the elders who are physically, sexually, and/or psychologically abused or neglected, and it may even raise their chances of dying. One study of more than 2,800 elders found that those who were abused or neglected were three times more likely than those who were not mistreated to die during the next thirteen years. This difference was found even after injury and chronic illness were taken into account (Horn, 1998).

A major reason for elder abuse seems to be stress. The adult children and other relatives who care for elders often find it an exhausting, emotionally trying experience, especially if the person they are helping needs extensive help with daily activities. Faced with this stress, elders' caregivers can easily snap and take out their frustrations with physical violence, emotional abuse, or neglect of care.

Senior Power: Older Americans as a Political Force

Older Americans often hold strong views on issues that affect them directly, such as Medicare and Social Security. In turn, politicians often work to win the older vote and shape their political stances accordingly.

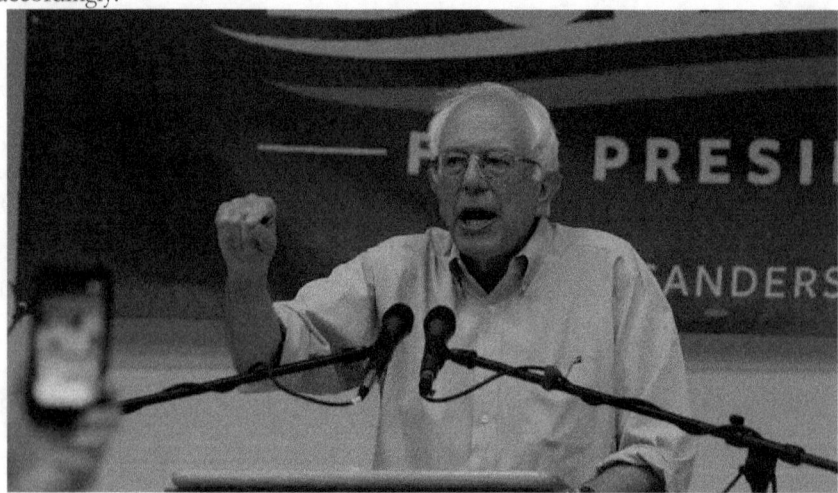

During the past few decades, older people have become more active politically on their own behalf.
Marc Nozell – Bernie Sanders – CC BY-NC 2.0.

To help address all the problems discussed in the preceding pages, several organizations have been established since the 1980s to act as interest groups in the political arena on behalf of older Americans (Walker, 2006). One of the most influential groups is the American Association of Retired Persons (AARP), which is open to people 50 or older. AARP provides travel and other discounts to its members and lobbies Congress and other groups extensively on elderly issues. Its membership numbers about 40 million, or 40 percent of the over-50 population. Some critics say AARP focuses too much on its largely middle-class membership's self-interests instead of working for more far-reaching economic changes that might benefit the older poor; others say

its efforts on Medicare, Social Security, and other issues do benefit the elderly from all walks of life. This controversy aside, AARP is an influential force in the political arena because of its numbers and resources.

A very different type of political organization of the elderly was the Gray Panthers, founded by the late Maggie Kuhn in 1970 (Kuhn, Long, & Quinn, 1991). Although this group has been less newsworthy since Kuhn's death in 1995, at its height it had some eighty-five local chapters across the nation and 70,000 members and supporters. A more activist organization than AARP and other lobbying groups for the elderly, the Gray Panthers took more liberal stances. For example, it urged the establishment of a national health-care service and programs to increase affordable housing for the elderly.

As older Americans have engaged the political process on their own behalf, critics have charged that programs for the elderly are too costly to the nation, that the elderly are better off than groups like AARP claim, and that new programs for the elderly will take even more money from younger generations and leave them insufficient funds for their own retirement many years from now. Their criticism, which began during the 1980s, is termed the generational equity argument (Williamson, McNamara, & Howling, 2003).

Advocates for the elderly say the generational equity critics exaggerate the financial well-being of older Americans and neglect the fact that many older Americans, especially women and those of color, are poor or near poor and thus need additional government aid. Anything we can do now to help the aged, they continue, will also help future generations of the elderly. As Lenard W. Kaye (1994, p. 346) observed in an early critique of the generational equity movement, "In the long run, all of us can expect to live into extended old age, barring an unexpected fatal illness or accident. To do injustice to our current generation of elders, by means of policy change, can only come back to haunt us as each and every one of us—children, young families, and working people—move toward the latter stages of the life course."

People Making a Difference

5. College Students Helping Senior Citizens

After Hurricane Irene swept up the East Coast in August 2011, many towns and cities faced severe flooding. One of these towns was Cranford, New Jersey, just southwest of Newark. Streets and hundreds of homes flooded, and many residents' belongings were ruined.

Union County College, which has campuses in Cranford and a few other towns, came to Cranford residents' aid. As the college president explained in late August, "Many of the town's residents are senior citizens. Even though the fall term won't begin until Sept. 1, we've still got a number of strong men and women on campus to help residents clear out their basements and help move whatever people needed moved."

Led by the dean of college life, a dozen or so students went house-to-house on a Cranford street that experienced the worst flooding to aid the town's senior citizens and younger ones as well. The dean later recalled, "Everyone we met was just so happy to see us there helping out. Sometimes they had plenty of work for us. Other times, they just smiled and said they were glad to know we cared."

A news report summarized the impact of the students' assistance: "In the coming weeks and months, Cranford residents will be able to recover what their town lost to Irene. But they may never forget the damage Irene caused, nor are they likely to forget how Union County College's students came to help them in their time of need." At a time of crisis, the staff and students of Union County College in the small town of Cranford, New Jersey, made a big difference in the lives of Cranford's senior citizens and younger residents alike.

Source: Cranford Chronicle, 2011

Key Takeaways

- The US elderly experience several health problems, including arthritis, high blood pressure, heart disease, hearing loss, vision problems, diabetes, and dementia.
- Nursing home care in the United States is very expensive and often substandard; neglect and abuse of nursing home residents is fairly common.
- Despite help from Social Security, many older Americans face problems of financial security.
- It is difficult to determine the actual extent of elder abuse, but elder abuse often has serious consequences for the health and lives of older Americans.
- During the last few decades, older Americans have been active in the political process on their own behalf and today are an important political force in the United States.

For Your Review

1. What do you think is the worst or most serious problem facing the US elderly? Explain your answer.

2. The text suggests that the lives of the US elderly would be improved if the United States were to adopt some of the policies and practices that other nations have for their elderly. Explain why you agree or disagree with this suggestion

References

Alzheimer's Association. (2009). *2009 Alzheimer's disease facts and figures.* Chicago, IL: Author.

Berger, E. D. (2009). Managing age discrimination: An examination of the techniques used when seeking employment. *The Gerontologist, 49*(3), 317–332.

Carr, D. (2010). Golden years? Poverty among older Americans. *Contexts, 9*(1), 62–63.

Cranford Chronicle. (2011, August 31). County College students help Cranford residents cleanup. *Cranford Chronicle.* Retrieved from http://www.nj.com/cranford/index.ssf/2011/2008/county_college_students_help_c.html
.

Crawthorne, A. (2008). *Elderly poverty: The challenge before us.* Washington, DC: Center for American Progress.

DeHart, D., Webb, J., & Cornman, C. (2009). Prevention of elder mistreatment in nursing homes: Competencies for direct-care staff. *Journal of Elder Abuse & Neglect, 21*(4), 360–378.

Edwards, M. (2007). As Good As It Gets: What Country Takes the Best Care of Its Older Citizens? In D. S. Eitzen (Ed.), *Solutions to Social Problems: Lessons from Other Societies*(4th ed., pp. 76–85). Boston, MA: Allyn & Bacon.

Federal Interagency Forum on Aging-Related Statistics. (2010). *Older Americans 2010: Key indicators of well-being.* Washington, DC: US Goverment Printing Office.

Gallo, W. T., Brand, J. E., Teng, H.-M., Leo-Summers, L., & Byers, A. L. (2009). Differential impact of involuntary job loss on physical disability among older workers: Does predisposition matter? *Research on Aging, 31*(3), 345–360.

Hartlapp, M., & Schmid, G. (2008). Labour market policy for "active ageing" in Europe: Expanding the options for retirement transitions. *Journal of Social Policy, 37*(3), 409–431.

Horn, D. (1998, August 17). Bad news on elder abuse. *Time*, p. 82.

Kaye, L. W. (1994). Generational equity: Pitting young against old. In J. Robert B. Enright (Ed.), *Perspectives in social gerontology* (pp. 343–347). Boston, MA: Allyn and Bacon.

Kerby, S. (2012). *Debunking poverty myths and racial stereotypes.* Washington, DC: Center for American Progress.

Kuhn, M., Long, C., & Quinn, L. (1991). *No stone unturned: The life and times of Maggie Kuhn.* New York, NY: Ballantine Books.

Leland, J. (2010, April 25). A graying population, a graying work force. *New York Times,* p. A14. National Center on Elder Abuse. (2010). *Why should I care about elder abuse?* Washington, DC: Author.

Ney, S. (2005). Active aging policy in Europe: Between path dependency and path departure. *Ageing International, 30,* 325–342.

Novak, M. (2012). *Issues in aging* (3rd ed.). Upper Saddle River, NJ: Pearson.
Roscigno, V. J. (2010). Ageism in the American workplace. *Contexts, 9*(1), 16–21.

Rowe, J. W., Berkman, L. F., Binstock, R., Boersch-Supan, A., Cacioppo, J., Carsternsen, L., et al. (2010). Policies and politics for an aging America. *Contexts, 9*(1), 22–27.

Sears, D. (2009, September 6). Myths busted on older workers' job performance. *TheLadders.* Retrieved from http://www.career-line.com/job-search-news/myths-busted-on-older-workersjob-performance/.

Walker, A. (2006). Aging and politics: An international perspective. In R. H. Binstock & L. K. George (Eds.), *Handbook of aging and the social sciences* (6th ed., pp. 338–358). New York, NY: Academic Press.

Williamson, J. B., McNamara, T. K., & Howling, S. A. (2003). Generational equity, generational interdependence, and the framing of the debate over social security reform. *Journal of Sociology and Social Welfare, 30*(3), 3–14.
Previous/next navigation

Previous: 6.4 Biological and Psychological Aspects of Aging

Next: 6.6 Reducing Ageism and Helping Older Americans

D. Health and Aging in the 21st Century

AUTHORS
Karen Davis

President's Message from 1999 Annual Report

The 20th century witnessed an explosion of medical science, industrialization, and economic progress, with resulting strides in life expectancy and economic prosperity. Will the 21st century bring even more dramatic gains in health and well-being? Or will the United States enter an era of limits on the capacity of the economy and the health system to assure a healthy and prosperous future for all? In particular, will we be able to sustain the health and economic security of older Americans as the baby boom generation reaches retirement after 2010?

To some extent, the future is up to us. Foundations, nonprofit organizations, business, labor, consumer groups, and civic and governmental leaders helped stimulate innovation and change throughout the 20th century, guided by a vision of a common cause in advancing social progress. The challenge for the 21st century is mobilizing the talent, creative thinking, and partnerships required to realize the potential that new advances in knowledge and information hold.

Demography Is Not Destiny

The specter of an aging population has spawned numerous government commissions and scores of legislative proposals to restructure Social Security and Medicare. Long-term projections abound: by one estimate, providing even the same level of benefits for a growing older population could double the share of the gross domestic product (GDP) now supporting those programs over the next 25 to 30 years, with Medicare outlays alone increasing from 2.5 percent of GDP today to 4.4 percent in 2025. Yet many such projections are based on assumptions about economic growth and trends in the health sector that may not be borne out in the long term.

In fact, demography is a relatively minor factor in determining the cost of social goods and services. Consider, for example, total health spending per capita. While it is true that people over age 65 generate health care expenditures about four times as high as those of younger people, aging occurs at a sufficiently slow rate that national levels of health spending are influenced much more by the overall structure of the health system and trends in care than by the age of the population. A cross-national examination finds no relationship between a nation's health spending and the percent of the population over age 65. In 1997, for example, the share of the American population over age 65 was 12.5 percent. In the same year, the elderly populations of the United Kingdom, France, Germany, and Japan were slightly above 16 percent—a rate the United States will reach only by 2020—yet all spent considerably less on health care as a percent of GDP. Further, health spending as a percent of GDP has been remarkably flat in these four countries over the last 15 years, a period during which health spending has risen rapidly in the United States.

There is no necessary link between high health spending and a large elderly population. France, Japan, the United Kingdom, and Germany all have more elderly (as a share of total population), yet all spend far less of total gross domestic product on health care.

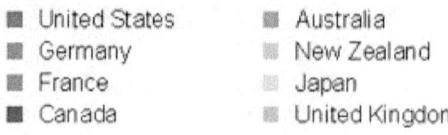

- ■ United States
- ■ Germany
- ■ France
- ■ Canada
- ■ Australia
- ■ New Zealand
- ■ Japan
- ■ United Kingdom

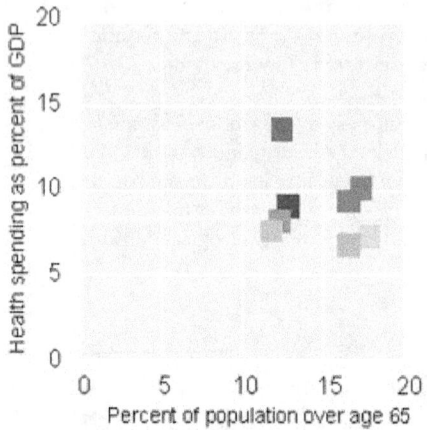

Source: G. Anderson and P. Hussey, *Health and Population Aging: A Multinational Comparison*, The Commonwealth Fund, October 1999.

Three major arguments suggest that current projections are uncertain and potentially misleading. First, changes in fertility and immigration rates are as important as changes in life expectancy in affecting future age distribution and the ratio of workers to retirees. While the fact that the U.S. population will grow older on average over the next 30 years is well recognized, there has been less attention to the implications of the growing diversity of the population and the changes in age distribution that may result. Racial and ethnic minorities now represent 28 percent of the U.S. population. By the year 2030, 40 percent of all Americans will belong to these groups. Economic, health, and social changes will be needed to respond to the changing makeup of the U.S. population and deserve much higher priority on the national agenda.

Second, the elderly of tomorrow will be different from those of today. Disability rates and nursing home admission rates have been declining. It is uncertain whether or not those trends will continue, but if they do, they will have a marked effect on the demands placed on the health system and the need for long-term care. Even without major breakthroughs in medical research or biotechnology, tomorrow's elderly will be healthier and better educated. Smoking rates have declined. Much more is known about measures that can prevent or delay the onset of functional impairment and contribute to successful aging. Efforts to change behavior and encourage healthier practices could significantly enhance the quality of life in old age.

Third, it is much more the case that economics, not demography, is destiny. Again, assumptions—in this case, about the rate of economic growth—weigh powerfully in future projections. From 1950 to 1997, real GDP grew 3.2 percent annually but slowed in the 1980s and early 1990s. In the last four years, however, economic growth has averaged 4 percent annually. The Congressional Budget Office assumes future economic growth will be 1.5 percent a year. If we experience 3 percent annual economic growth over the next 30 years, average GDP per capita will be almost double what it would be if economic growth were 1 percent ($64,637 as opposed to $33,491, in constant 1998 dollars). Similarly, government expenditures as a percent of GDP could range from 32 percent in 2030, assuming 3 percent real growth, to 61 percent, assuming 1 percent real growth. The nation's capacity to finance health care and assure economic security for the old, while also allowing for higher private consumption and savings, will hinge critically on the future of the economy.

Different assumptions about the future rate of economic growth produce very different pictures of what our society will look like in 30 years—and what our nation can afford.

■ Assuming 1% growth
■ Assuming 3% growth

Total government expenditures as percent of GDP

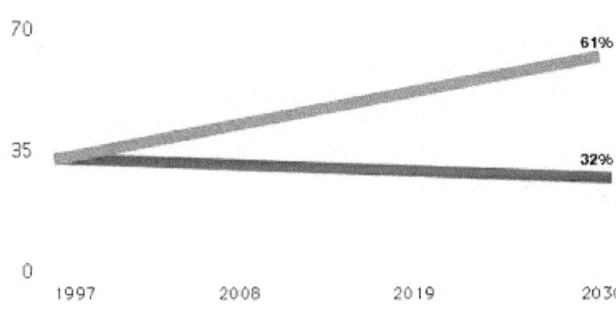

Source: R. Friedland and L. Summer, *Demography Is Not Destiny*, National Academy on an Aging Society, Gerontological Society of America, January 1999.

Averages conceal important variations among older people. Over the last two decades, the incomes of working families have become more unequal, and pension and retiree health benefits have covered a declining proportion of workers. Thus, some of tomorrow's elderly will enter retirement in a much less secure financial position than others. Illness or the early death of a spouse can affect economic security, especially for widows in retirement, since single women have much lower incomes on average than do other older Americans. Out-of-pocket medical expenses not covered by Medicare or supplemental insurance also place a major financial burden on the chronically ill.

Policies implemented today that promote economic growth, expand opportunities for older people to use their skills in meaningful work and volunteer activities, share economic prosperity more broadly, protect against the financial losses inflicted by uncovered medical bills for both young and old, improve access to high-quality health care, and promote healthy behaviors will all have significant implications for the future. Our destiny is in our hands; it is not determined by demography alone.

Medicare: Myth versus Reality

The United States is unique among countries in financing health care for the elderly through a governmental program while financing care for working families largely through employer-sponsored health insurance. Thus, a shift in the percentage of the population over age 65 inevitably leads to a shift in the share of total health spending financed by taxes. By 2025, Medicare beneficiaries will be 20.6 percent of the population, up from 13.8 percent in 1998. Concern about the higher taxes needed to finance this change has focused attention on the "Medicare crisis." While it is important to plan for an aging population and debate policy alternatives, myths and confusion currently cloud the discussion.

Two-thirds of Medicare beneficiaries have health problems, low incomes, or both. Either factor can make it very difficult to pay for health care costs, such as prescription drugs, that are not covered by Medicare.

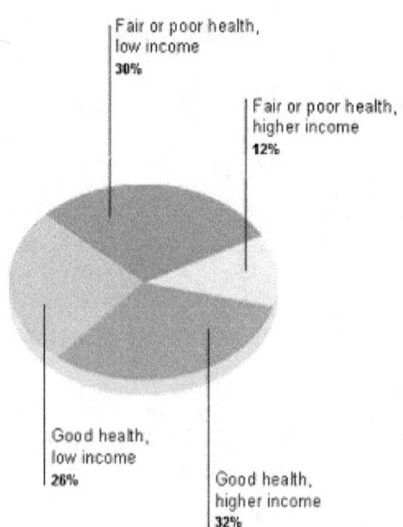

Fair or poor health, low income
30%

Fair or poor health, higher income
12%

Good health, low income
26%

Good health, higher income
32%

Note: Fair or poor health includes disabled under age 65. Low income includes those with incomes at or below 200% of the federal poverty level.

Source: Kaiser/Commonwealth 1997 Survey of Medicare Beneficiaries, December 1998.

The first major myth is that Medicare beneficiaries are affluent. The reality is that, although incomes vary for older people as they do for younger, most Medicare beneficiaries have modest incomes. Three-quarters have incomes under $25,000, and more than half of women on Medicare have incomes under $10,000. A more accurate portrait of a typical Medicare beneficiary is old, sick, and poor or near poor. A survey by the Henry J. Kaiser Family Foundation and the Fund found that only one-third of Medicare beneficiaries enjoy good health and have incomes above 200 percent of the federal poverty level.

The second myth is that Medicare benefits are too generous, or that the amounts beneficiaries are required to contribute are too low. In fact, Medicare benefits have not improved markedly in the last 35 years. Today, 95 percent of the major health plans offered to employees by medium or large firms cover prescription drugs, but Medicare does not. For the most part, long-term care is not covered either. Medicare's hospital deductible is $768, compared with $201 (in 1998 dollars) when the program started in 1966; the Part B annual premium is $546, compared with $181 at the program's outset.

As a result, most Medicare beneficiaries, unlike workers covered by employer-financed coverage, need supplemental insurance. Only 34 percent of Medicare beneficiaries now get retiree health benefits through their former employers, and this share will decline in the future. For those who must purchase supplemental coverage, the typical premium for a policy purchased individually is approximately $1,250 annually. These premiums and non-covered services account for the fact that the typical Medicare beneficiary pays $2,600 for health care each year, or nearly 20 percent of income. By contrast, non-elderly families spend about 8 percent of income on out-of-pocket health care costs. Any proposal to shift more costs from working years to retirement would further widen his disparity and add to the savings required to finance retirement.

Today's Medicare beneficiaries pay significant sums for their care—far more than when the program started in 1966. Including the cost of prescription drugs, supplemental coverage, and other non-covered costs, they spend an average of $2,600 annually.

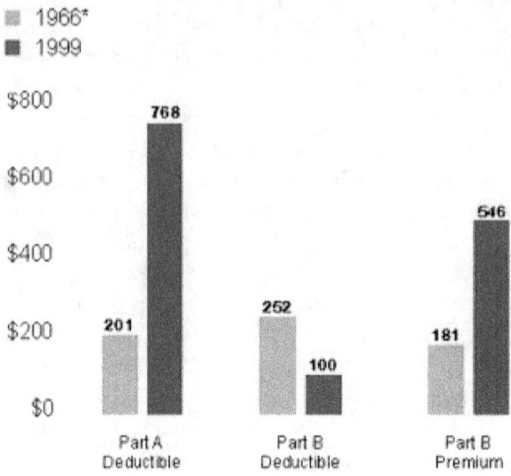

■ 1966*
■ 1999

*1966 figures are in 1998 dollars

Source: Calculated by K. Davis with data from the 1998 *Green Book*, U.S. House of Representatives, and HCFA, Office of the Actuary.

The high expenses incurred by Medicare beneficiaries, coupled with their modest incomes, make it clear that the potential to finance health spending for an aging population through higher beneficiary contributions is quite limited. Projections indicate that by 2025 Medicare beneficiaries will be spending 29 percent of income on their own health care. For those who have serious health problems or below-average incomes, an even higher share of income will be devoted to health care. Although a small minority of future retirees will enter old age with substantial savings and income from pensions and investments, those same individuals will have contributed more to Medicare while working (since there is no longer a ceiling on earnings subject to the Part A payroll tax) and will continue to contribute more through income taxes that help finance Medicare Part B.

The third myth is that Medicare is inefficient and costly, and that the "Medicare crisis" could be averted if the program were reformed to rely more on managed care and market competition among private insurers. In fact, Medicare has a history of remarkable administrative efficiency. Its administrative costs average less than 2 percent, compared with 10-15 percent in employer group coverage and 30-50 percent in individual private health insurance. Medicare expenses per beneficiary have risen at the same rate over the last 25 years as private health insurance costs per covered person for comparable benefits. Given the sharp curtailment of payments to managed care plans, hospitals, physicians, and other health care providers as specified in the 1997 Balanced Budget Act, Medicare spending is projected to grow much more slowly than private insurance costs over the next five years.

Out-of-pocket health spending consumes nearly 20 percent of the income of the typical elderly American today. That rate could reach 29 percent in 2025, even without increases in beneficiary contributions for Medicare.

Percent of annual income spent on health care by a typical elderly Medicare beneficiary

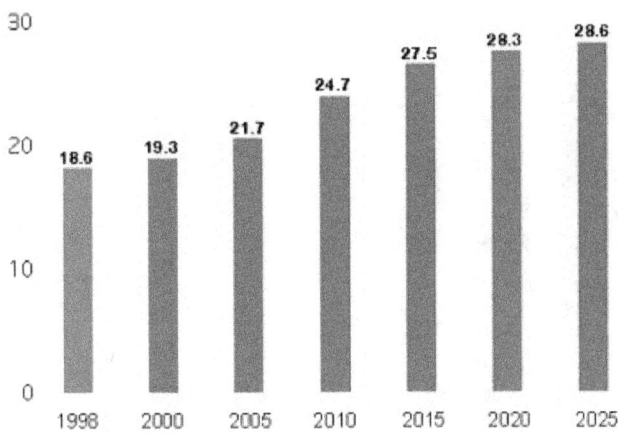

Source: M. Moon, *Growth in Medicare Spending: What will Beneficiaries Pay?*
The Commonwealth Fund, May 1999.

Medicare already makes about 300 managed care plans available to beneficiaries, and about 14 percent of beneficiaries—6 million—belong to those plans. The value of this option is still in question. The Medicare managed care industry is experiencing considerable turbulence, and some health plans have left selected markets, raised premiums, or trimmed benefits. Current estimates indicate that Medicare pays about 6 percent more for each beneficiary enrolled in managed care than it does for those who remain in traditional Medicare. Efforts to test competitive bidding or other incentives to reduce costs have encountered considerable resistance. New methods of paying plans on the basis of health risks have not yet been adopted, and the first open enrollment season—during which beneficiaries were supposed to be informed more fully about their choices—met with only mixed success.

One proposal under consideration, called "premium support," would further "privatize" Medicare. Under this approach the federal government, rather than paying directly for care through traditional Medicare or managed care plans, would contribute a fixed sum that beneficiaries could apply toward the cost of their care. Beneficiaries would be responsible for the difference between the actual cost and the government's contribution.

Under the proposed "premium support" approach, the federal government would contribute a fixed sum toward the care of each Medicare beneficiary. The result could be even higher out-of-pocket spending by elderly Americans.

Percent of annual income spent on health care by a beneficiary in traditional Medicare

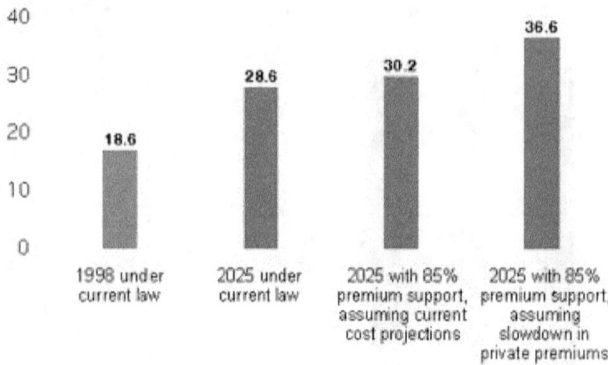

Source: M. Moon, *Restructuring Medicare: Impacts on Beneficiaries*, The Commonwealth Fund, May 1999.

The Health Care Financing Administration has estimated (based in part on a proposal to set the federal contribution at 88 percent of the median private managed care premium) that premium support and other provisions such as raising the age of eligibility to 67 could help save about 11 percent of Medicare outlays over the next 30 years. Yet most of these "savings" are costs shifted to beneficiaries. Under the proposal, beneficiaries would pay $5,000 per person in 2025 (in 1998 dollars), or about 30 percent of income, for their own care. Savings also depend on the untested assumption that competition among plans would lead to lower premiums over time. And, if private managed care premiums were indeed to fall, the cost to beneficiaries of remaining in traditional Medicare could rise substantially, consuming 37 percent of income by 2025.

Options for restructuring Medicare are likely to be the subject of intense debate over the next few years. The Medicare Part A hospital fund will be exhausted in 2015. The absence of an immediate deadline for action has the advantage of permitting a more thorough discussion of how best to finance health care for an aging population in the 21st century. It also grants time to assess the validity of a more optimistic view of economic growth, the progress of medical research, and the health of an aging population.

The optimists call for dedicating a portion of the federal budget surplus to Medicare and expanding benefits to include prescription drugs. Savings would be achieved by extending limits on payments to health care providers beyond 2002, when the Balanced Budget Act provisions expire. Some additional payments by beneficiaries would be required through partial premiums, coinsurance for prescription drug coverage, and other measures. Also, steps might be taken to restructure financial contributions from beneficiaries to provide greater protection to the poor and sick while collecting premiums from those with more substantial incomes.

Close monitoring, solid information about options, and addressing some of the factors that undermine health and economic security in retirement could all contribute to a healthier and more prosperous nation in the 21st century. The Fund will continue to advance understanding of the issues by projecting trends, simulating policy options, and analyzing specific proposals through its Program on Medicare's Future.

Long-Term Care and End-of-Life Care

The aging of the population also has implications for long-term and end-of-life care. Under the current system, with Medicaid the predominant source of payment for nursing home care, many older Americans face the undignified prospect of exhausting their savings to the point of impoverishment before qualifying for assistance with long-term care expenses. Until our nation adopts a financing system capable of accommodating the needs of Americans across the income spectrum, the personal and financial issues associated with long-term care can only grow more difficult.

Recent estimates indicate that the number of elderly people with long-term care needs will rise substantially, from 8.7 million today to 12 million by 2030. The services required are diverse, ranging from care in a nursing home to personal care at home. A year in a nursing home costs around $40,000 on average, and twice that in some states. Medicare, Medicaid, and other government programs (such as the Veterans Administration) cover about two-thirds of the nation's $115 billion annual spending on long-term care. About 28 percent of those costs are paid directly by families; only 7 percent are covered by private insurance.

Projections of future national spending on long-term care for the elderly indicate continued growth as more baby boomers reach age 65 and more elderly live to be 85 years or older. Total spending is expected to rise to $346 billion by 2040 (in 2000 dollars), of which two-thirds would pay for nursing home care. Rising expenditures for long-term care have important implications for the Medicaid program. By 2040, Medicaid outlays for long-term care are expected to reach $125 billion (in 2000 dollars), up from $43 billion in the year 2000, and the projected financial burden on families is also substantial.

Yet most people's fears about long-term care are not primarily financial. Rather, the dearth of high-quality care options that are responsive to the preferences of patients and their families is more troubling. The quality of personal care in nursing homes is frequently deficient, the standards that do exist are often poorly enforced, and families have little information on which to make informed decisions. Not surprisingly, most people would prefer to be cared for at home, but finding and paying for qualified home care can be an insurmountable task.

Developing a better approach to financing and delivering long-term care services is a major challenge facing health care leaders and policy officials—and one that has received very little attention. We enter the 21st century without a basic system of financing long-term care, adequate standards to govern quality of care, or a shared understanding of the best approaches to providing care that is sensitive to patient and family preferences. The Fund is helping to build a base of knowledge through its support for quality measurements in nursing homes and dissemination of information to those who can act on it, from family members to state nursing home inspectors.

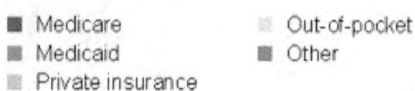

Total spending on long-term care will multiply in the coming decades. By 2040, Medicaid's share could be $125 billion, while the cost to families—in out-of-pocket spending and private insurance premiums—could reach $132 million.

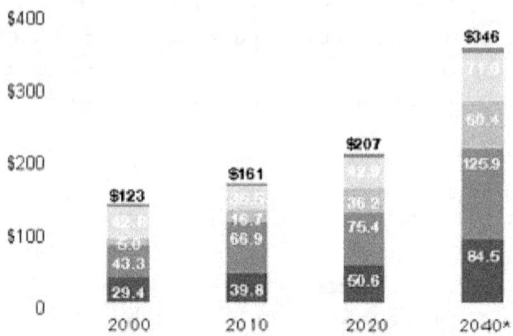

■ Medicare   ▨ Out-of-pocket
■ Medicaid   ■ Other
▨ Private insurance

Billions, in 2000 dollars

$400

$300 $346
                                                  71.9
                                                  60.4
$200 $207   125.9
                      $161   42.9
            $123   16.7   36.2
$100   42.8   66.9   75.4
            5.8   84.5
            43.3   39.8   50.6
    0   29.4   50.6
           2000   2010   2020   2040*

*2040 payer distribution based on distribution in 2020

Source: Projections from the Congressional Budget Office, March 1999.

Yet the experience of other countries is heartening. Denmark, for example, cut nursing home use per person over age 67 by 27 percent between 1982 and 1996; it also provides universal home care, using salaried nurses and trained aides employed by municipal governments. The cost to government of this publicly financed system is approximately 2.3 percent of GDP, although the percentage of elderly is already higher in Denmark than it is projected to be in the United States in 20 years' time. This and other potentially valuable lessons emerged from an international symposium sponsored by the Fund in October 1999 on cross-national approaches to financing and delivering quality long-term care.

Care for the terminally ill is also a much-neglected issue. A survey of terminally ill patients and family caregivers supported by the Nathan Cummings Foundation and the Fund finds that the current system often fails to meet the needs of families. Burdens on caregivers are substantial, and uncovered expenses can be financially devastating, even to middle class families. These findings shed some light on approaches that could make end-of-life care more responsive to the preferences of patients and families and on the need for greater support for family members and improved financial protection for services such as prescription drugs.

Opportunities to Promote Healthier Old Age

One obvious but undervalued strategy for addressing the aging of the population is to become much more methodical about understanding and promoting healthier old age. This is the fundamental premise of the Beeson Scholars Program, supported by the John A. Hartford Foundation, donor friends of the Alliance for Aging Research, and the Fund, which seeks to increase medical research on aging and attract physician scientists to the field. The program is expanding the pool of talented young investigators committed to research on aging, while also building a network capable of employing that knowledge for practical purposes.

Many older women fail to get preventive care that can help them stay healthy and active into old age. The problem is most acute among women over 65.

■ Ages 50–64
■ Age 65 and over

Percent of women

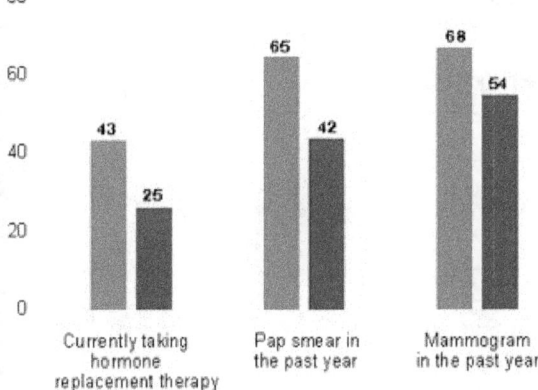

Source: 1998 Commonwealth Fund Survey of Women's Health.

Indeed, much more could be done to apply what is already known to improve the health and quality of life of older people. At Yale-New Haven Hospital, for example, a project funded in part by the National Institute on Aging, the Retirement Research Foundation, local funders, and the Fund sought to prevent delirium among older, at-risk hospitalized patients. An evaluation showed that the project succeeded in reducing the incidence of delirium by 40 percent, at a savings in hospital charges of $2,000 per patient. The intervention, known as the Elder Life Program, uses trained volunteers to walk patients three times a day, help them remain oriented, provide cognitive stimulation, enhance sleeping at night through relaxation techniques, and identify and correct visual and hearing impairment. The challenge is to make this a standard of care for all hospitals.

Missed opportunities to prevent morbidity and mortality exist for all ages, but the situation is particularly serious for older people. A RAND study supported by the Fund found that only about half of people with hypertension have their condition controlled, only half of diabetics receive regular eye exams, and only one-tenth of people with a current depressive disorder receive antidepressant medications.

Inadequate preventive care is common. Although the risk of cancer is highest among older people, older women are less likely to receive regular mammograms and Pap smears than younger women. Almost half of women over 65 fail to get a regular mammogram, and more than half do not get a regular Pap smear. Rates of regular colon cancer screening are also quite low for this age group: 26 percent of women and 41 percent of men. The Commonwealth Fund 1998 Survey of Women's Health found that only 47 percent of women over age 65 are very familiar with osteoporosis and only 57 percent take calcium supplements. Hormone replacement therapy has significant benefits in reducing risks of heart disease and osteoporosis, but only 25 percent of older women receive such therapy, and only 26 percent receive any counseling from their physicians about this option.

Differences in receipt of basic services such as influenza vaccines or eye exams show that racial disparities persist even after age 65, when all Americans become eligible for Medicare.

Percent of Medicare beneficiaries* who received influenza vaccine in the past year, 1996

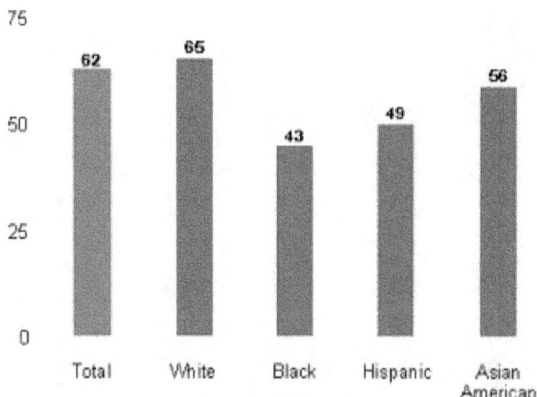

*Age 65 and older, community-dwelling

Source: K. Collins, A. Hall, and C. Neuhaus, *U.S. Minority Health: A Chartbook*, The Commonwealth Fund, 1999.

Minority elderly are even more at risk. Only 43 percent of black elderly received an influenza vaccine in the past year, compared with 65 percent of white elderly. Minority elderly Medicare beneficiaries are less likely to receive specialized services, such as angioplasty, coronary artery bypass graft surgery, or hip fracture repair.

If we are serious about assuring a healthy and prosperous old age for all, we will need to adopt a more systematic approach to assuring high-quality care and applying what is known about health-enhancing and preventive measures. The Fund is contributing to this effort by supporting the development of Health Employer Data Information Set (HEDIS) quality measures, which are used to assess the performance of managed care plans. New categories will include, for example, physician counseling for postmenopausal women on the benefits and risks of hormone replacement therapy. The Fund also supports efforts to extend innovative models, such as the program at Yale-New Haven Hospital. But these are just a beginning. Until we as a nation make prevention and quality of care a top priority, we will continue to miss opportunities to enhance the quality of life in old age.

Future Challenges

Continued strong economic growth holds the key to a prosperous future for all Americans. The government, business, and nonprofit sectors have all contributed to the most recent upturn in productivity and, working in concert, can assure its continuation in the 21st century. Low unemployment provides opportunities for more Americans—minorities, single mothers, immigrants, people with disabilities, and older people—to contribute to and share in economic prosperity.

A key to continued growth is investment early in life to assure that all children grow up healthy and productive. Along with more than 70 cofounders, the Fund has invested in a new approach to pediatric care called Healthy Steps, which provides parents with information and services to promote the cognitive, behavioral, and social development of their infants from birth to age three. This and other innovations can do much to build a strong labor force by assuring that all children reach school age ready and able to learn.

But older Americans can also continue to contribute in meaningful ways to work, family, and community life. The Fund's earlier Americans Over 55 at Work Program demonstrated that many older people are ready, able, and willing to work but lack opportunities because of deeply held biases about the adaptability and productivity of older workers. Older people can also contribute significantly through volunteer activities. A Fund-supported survey found that mentors can help guide young people into further education and productive careers. The Elder Life Program to prevent delirium also demonstrated a valuable role for volunteers. Using volunteers more creatively in ospitals, nursing homes, and other settings could enhance quality of life and reduce the cost to society of health and long-term care.

Shared economic prosperity is also essential to a better future. Parents who earn a decent wage can provide more opportunities for their children to develop to their full potential. Families with good health insurance are more likely to get care that prevents illness and disability and are better protected from the financial burdens of uncovered medical bills. The Fund's new Task Force on the Future of Health Insurance for Working Americans is dedicated explicitly to the needs of uninsured and low wage workers. We all have a common cause in assuring that people enter retirement in good health and economically secure, not sick, and poor. Paying for health and long-term care for an aging population will be easier if tomorrow's Medicare beneficiaries and workers are well prepared.

Another important goal is to assure that the American health care system is driven to achieve excellence. The preoccupation in the last quarter century with slowing the growth of health care costs has shifted attention away from technological innovation and high-quality care. Indeed, the Fund's Task Force on Academic Health Centers has shown that managed care is eroding the nation's medical research capacity and undermining the social missions of academic health centers. Yet, over the last half of the 20th century, the greatest gains in health, life expectancy, and functioning have come from advances in medical science and improvements in specialized care, whether drug discoveries or new techniques in cardiac, cataract, orthopedic, and other types of surgery.

Leaders in medicine and health care institutions are increasingly frustrated by constraints on their ability to provide the kind of care that patients want and need, and by a reward system that appears not to value excellence in patient care or innovation. A medical practice that spends time on patient education — whether about diabetes, hormone replacement therapy, or child development — must do so at an economic loss. The Fund's Survey of Physician Experiences with Managed Care found that two-fifths of physicians say they have less ability than they did three years ago to make decisions they think are right for their patients. An equal proportion report that they are spending less time with patients.

The United States spends more on health care per capita than any other country — by a factor of two. Incentives to improve efficiency and reduce inappropriate or unnecessary care are important. But equally important is a health system that rewards physicians whose patients have their hypertension or diabetes well controlled and understand the options available to them to reduce the risk of future disease and disability. Advances in information technology hold great promise for engaging patients in their own care decisions, improving physician-patient communication, promoting healthy behavior, feeding individual and comparative information back to providers, and preventing medical errors through "real time" information systems that are readily accessible. We are just at the beginning of our ability to tap information technology as a powerful tool to transform American medicine.

Compared with these challenges, financing health and long-term care for an aging population should be relatively straightforward. Efforts to date have searched for a painless magic bullet, a cure-all that would permit more
comprehensive benefits, reduce costs to beneficiaries, impose no new taxes, and maintain rates of payment to hospitals, physicians, and other providers of services. Managed care and the privatization of Medicare are not panaceas.

Medicare was enacted in 1965 because private insurers would not provide adequate coverage for American retirees. Since then, it has served a very important function by covering all, regardless of income or health status. As the program is updated, this essential feature should be protected. Fortunately, a stronger-than-anticipated economy, along with the Balanced Budget Act of 1997—which tightened payment rates to health care providers—have assured Medicare's solvency for the next 15 years. This reprieve should give the nation an opportunity to explore a range of realistic, long-term options to assure the health of older Americans in the 21st century and promote excellence in care, as Medicare has done so well during the last third of the 20th century.

There is no comparable base for building a 21st century approach to long-term care financing. Today, Medicaid is the major source of financing for nursing home and home- and communitybased care for those who cannot care for themselves, but it is available only after all savings are exhausted. Quality of care is a serious concern: despite some recent improvements, such as reductions in the use of restraints, instances of substandard care are far too common. More fundamentally, families have no assurance that there are choices available that will permit their family members to receive kind, loving care in the twilight of life. Other countries have already grappled with many of these issues, in part because they have already experienced the aging that will overtake the United States in the next few decades. Cross-national exchange of experiences affords some promise of building on proven models of care.

Advances have made health care more patient-centered. Through the work of the Fundsupported Picker Institute and others, hospitals now routinely survey discharged patients about their experiences, and consumer assessment of managed care plans has become standard practice. Employers and consumers are beginning to use quality information to make more informed choices, but to a very limited extent. Feeding back information to plans and providers appears to be having a growing impact. And some purchasers (whether employers or managed care plans) are beginning to develop incentives to reward excellence. It is an opportune time to begin to take the concepts of patient-centered care into the arenas of long-term care and care of the dying. Listening to patients and families is an important first step.

It is sometimes said that only in America is death viewed as an option. But the possibility of a healthier, longer life may become a reality in the 21st century. Advances in medical research and biotechnology may unlock the secrets of disease and, through gene therapy and other techniques, eliminate some of the major causes of disability and premature mortality. No one can predict the future course of health and disability, but much can be done today to make sure that what is known to be beneficial is more broadly available.

No other sector of the American economy would tolerate the high rate of failure that prevails in American health care: the children who are not immunized, the adolescents who begin risky behaviors that have lifetime health consequences, the women who are not familiar with the steps they can take to reduce their risks of osteoporosis and heart disease, the men and women whose cancer is not detected at an early stage when the promise of cure is high, and the elderly whose hypertension, diabetes, and depression are not controlled. We can do better as a nation. And in doing better, we can lighten the burden on families, increase the quality of life, and contribute to increased labor productivity and economic growth.

Achieving these goals will take a wholehearted commitment to excellence for all. **We cannot continue with a health system that excludes some of our people because they lack health insurance or because of their race, ethnicity, or income. Nor can we continue to be blind to shortcomings in the present system.** Rather, we need to harness all the resources at our Command—including the potential of new information technology, visionary health care leaders, and dedicated health professionals—to improve the performance of the health system and reduce missed opportunities. These are just some of the priorities the Fund hopes to address through programs to improve health care services in general and the health of minority Americans, the elderly, and children in particular.

It is an exciting challenge, worthy of a new century. In embracing that challenge, the Fund pledges to draw on its historic strengths: a commitment to social progress, a tradition of scientific inquiry, partnership with others who share common concerns, effective use of communications, and mobilizing talented people to take on the challenges ahead. This *Annual Report* sets forth the Fund's efforts over the past year and outlines the major programs through which we hope to tackle the tasks ahead.

PUBLICATION DETAILS

Health and Aging in the 21st Century, Karen Davis, PH.D., March 3, 2000, The Commonwealth Fund

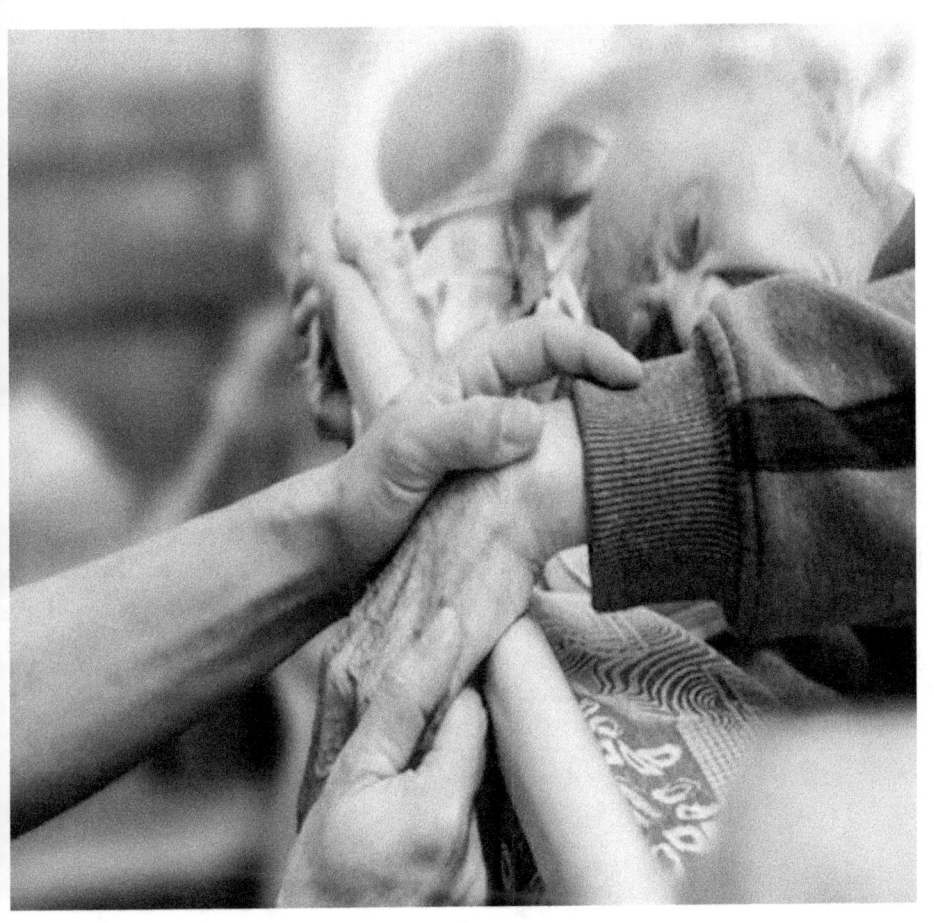

ABOUT THE AUTHOR

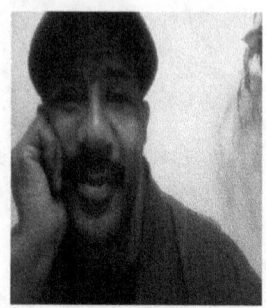

L. D. Peden (aka/Chibuzo Emem Onyejeweke) is a married writer, fitness enthusiast, and motorcycle fanatic living in Maryland. He is the owner and CEO of JoKeJa Books & Publishing, LLC. A former journalist, who has written professionally for *The AFRO American*, *The Prince George's Post*, *The Laurel Leader, Prudence International Magazine,* and various other publications. He worked for eight years in the healthcare industry, receiving his licensing and certification as a Geriatric Nursing Assistant in 2009. He is a graduate of Washington Adventist University, with a Bachelor of Fine Arts (BA), in Journalism/Pre-Law, and can be contacted at jokejabooks@gmail.com.